CW01391255

A Silent Tsunami

A Silent Tsunami

Swimming Against the Tide of my Mother's Dementia

ANTHEA ROWAN

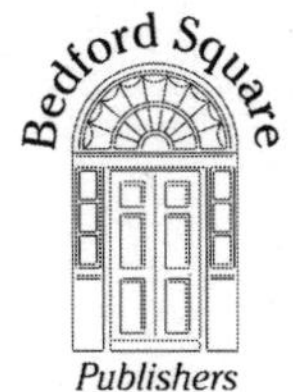

First published in the UK in 2024 by Bedford Square Publishers Ltd,
London, UK

bedfordsquarepublishers.co.uk
@bedsqpublishers

A CIP catalogue record for this book is available from the British Library.

ISBN
978-1-83501-057-0 (Hardback)
978-1-83501-058-7 (eBook)

2 4 6 8 10 9 7 5 3 1

Typeset in 12 on 15.65pt Bembo Std
by Avocet Typeset, Bideford, Devon, EX39 2BP
Printed and bound in Great Britain by
CPI Group (UK) Ltd, Croydon CR0 4YY

For Mum. Who forgot who I was.
For my children. Whom I hope I never forget.

Contents

Prologue 9

Chapter 1: Storm Warning 13

Chapter 2: Deep Blue 31

Chapter 3: Rip Tide 53

Chapter 4: The Octopus Mother 75

Chapter 5: Learning to Swim 115

Chapter 6: Salt as Cure 139

Chapter 7: Adrift 169

Chapter 8: Charting New Depths 179

Chapter 9: A Rising Tide 211

Chapter 10: A Silent Tsunami 237

Chapter 11: Drowning not Waving 273

Chapter 12: An Ebbing Tide 293

Epilogue 329

Prologue

February 2022

Sometimes my mother thinks she lives on a ship. She doesn't. She lives with me, a long way from the sea. Or any significant body of water. And yet: 'Am I on a ship?'

'No, Ma. You're high on dry land.'

'Oh.'

I can't tell if she's disappointed. But I can tell she doesn't believe me; she inches towards the window, pulls the curtain back and slyly surveys the fields and trees that spill in every direction, hoping – I know – to provide the evidence that I am wrong.

'What's that then? If it's not the sea?'

'Those are hills, Mum. But they look blue in this light,' I add.

(Not blue enough to be the sea – but blue enough that I can excuse them as something other than hills.)

Sometimes Mum asks, 'When should I start packing?'

'Packing?'

'Yes, packing: to get off the ship when we dock?'

Occasionally she will tell me about the person who used to share her 'cabin' with her.

'I miss her,' she says, sounding mournful, and then, brightening, 'but at least I have more space now.'

My mother has slept in a room of her own for almost forty years. There has always been space.

The first time I heard my mother reference her ship was after a dream, a dream so compelling it spilled into her consciousness.

That night she *was* near the sea, holidaying with me. Ocean waves were not seen in the distant undulations of blue-green hills, they were pounding the beach for real right outside her window. Perhaps the surf drummed its beat into her sleep and brought her dream to life.

Back then, excuses were easier.

My mother's dream was so persuasive it had her up and out of bed; that night she was living the dream for real. In her half-awake-state, she moved from her bed to her bathroom and pulled its sticky door tight-shut behind her.

Concerned when she did not appear to join me in our usual habit of early morning tea the next morning, or answer my voice when I called, I went to check on her and heard banging and angry tones from behind the stuck-closed door. I tugged it open and was immediately face to face with her as she dropped the fists she'd held aloft to thump on the door again.

She was furious.

'Why did you lock me in?' she shouted.

'Lock you in?'

'Yes. Why did you lock me in? In my cabin? I've been here all night!'

Her voice is high and she gestures around the tiny bathroom with impatient, frustrated hand-flapping as if I should know exactly what she is ranting about.

'But I didn't, Mum. Why would I? And anyway, this is your *bathroom*.'

Slowly, she collects herself and takes in my expression and

her familiar surroundings, her head turning as she scopes the room – her things, her toothbrush, her toilet bag. I see realisation begin to illuminate her face.

'I must have been dreaming,' she says, 'I was on a ship, you see. I was trying to escape, but I couldn't get out. I gave up in the end and made myself a bed on the floor,' and I notice a pitiful little nest of towels in the corner of the shower. 'I must have been dreaming,' she says again. As if to confirm this fact to herself.

'I'm sorry, Mum. Let me bring you tea on the veranda,' and I take her hand and lead her outside.

She settles into a chair, patting the dog's head and cooing good mornings to her.

It is only when I return with her mug of tea that I notice the back of her head; her white hair is painted pink with blood that has dried and matted it into dark clumps.

'Mum! Your head,' and I rush to examine it. There is a deep gash, gaping wide and still seeping. I already know this will need sutures.

Later, when I try to understand where, how, this has happened, I will find a small blood splatter against the bathroom tiles and conclude that she clambered onto the loo to try to reach a window – in that somnolent endeavour to escape – and fell backwards.

'Oh,' she says, her fingers rising to probe the damage, 'I must have fallen. When I was trying to get off the ship, I must have fallen,' and she smiles ruefully at me.

I held my mother's Dementia at the arm's length afforded by denial for as long as I could. But it is plain now: she has boarded that ship of her dreams and she is adrift. The changes in her tug like something unmoored. Soon she'll float clean off the edge of my horizons.

'Are you *sure* I'm not on a ship?' she asks, again, still at the window, studying the ripple of distant hills.

'I'm sure, Mum,' I say, and then, 'Come, let me help you down the steps.'

And I hold out my hand for her to grasp and I lead her down to the garden so that we can both feel the earth beneath our feet.

Chapter 1: Storm Warning

December 2019

When I go down the beach at dawn, the night's high tide has swept it clean. I look across the sand before I walk to the waterline and hesitate briefly, reluctant to sully its smoothness with my footprints.

It's as if yesterday's story – a story of families who played here, built sandcastles, threw towels down to lie on, chucked a ball for a dog, flew a kite – has been rubbed out. Battlements and towers cast of bucket and spade and strung with a bunting of seaweed have been levelled. Holes dug have been filled. Evidence of hundreds of feet erased. Today the beach will write a new story on sand clean as a fresh page.

I walk across this clean-slate-sand now and wade into the water. I look back. And there it is: the first line of my story for the day, my even tread in shallow indentations down to the shore: a clue to how I began my morning.

I break the surface easily as I swim out, I can feel the power of every stroke, propelling me forward, faster, further; further than I mean to. I'm startled when I stop and roll onto my back and see the smallness of the house on the cliff. I have swum until I am just a dot if you're sitting up there, on the veranda, where we will sit later. Over breakfast somebody might say, 'You went out miles today, I could only just see you: a dot on the horizon.'

I float for a bit, watch the sun peel the sky bright blue then swim back to the shore. I walk back up the beach towards the house. I gather up the towel I left slung on a branch and rub myself dry. I look back at the sea as I do – and there it is: another sentence in the sand. Another day; another story.

★ ★ ★

The evening my mother forgot who I was – who I am – was just like the one that had come before, and the one before that. Weeks of evenings all alike. I puzzled about that later. Why *that* evening? Why so sudden? So that at lunchtime she knew I was her daughter and by nightfall she didn't.

Six hours later. That's all it took. All the time it took for her view of me to become something else entirely, and for mine of the sea to change completely: the jade and green of the sun-dappled sandy shallows of a low tide to be drowned out by heaving, high black water.

A quite different story would be written on the beach the next day: I wouldn't swim the next morning.

I say to myself afterwards and often, over and over, 'I'll never, ever forget what that felt like; I'll never, ever forget this day.'

And I say to my children, who witness my devastation at my mother's forgetting who I am, and begin to worry that one day they'll experience the same: 'I'll never ever forget you, I promise.'

But how do you know?

You don't.

★ ★ ★

As one of a panel discussion on Dementia entitled 'Alzheimer's: Like a Tsunami, by the time you see it, it is too late,' Professor Craig Ritchie, CEO and Founder of Scottish Brain Sciences and Professor of Brain Health and Neurodegenerative Medicine at the University of St Andrews, was quoted as saying, 'We talk about there being a long, silent period of this disease before Dementia develops, but it's only silent because we are not listening properly.'

I wasn't listening, and by the time I heard the roar of the turn of a tide, the rise of a wave, it was too late to do anything.

* * *

The veranda faces the ocean and the east so that at dawn, when the sun pokes long fingers beneath the eaves, and pinches, we sit with spines straight against the back wall. We huddle in mean shade and drink tea.

Mum fans herself impatiently with an old envelope somebody has used as a shopping list so that I can see what was bought – tomato sauce, baking powder, bath soap – and what was not (brown rice and cotton wool remain unchecked). Mum, fresh from an autumnal Ireland, complains regularly about our East African equatorial heat.

When we sit out here later though, at dusk, at the tipping end of the day, we draw our chairs from the morning's back wall out onto the lawn, so that we can catch the breeze and watch the sea and the sky.

Some evenings, on a rising tide, the surf, a frill of white lace at its throat, runs up the sand chasing ghost crabs and obliterating the tread of their small weight in a single lick. Over and over that story is told: one minute the sand is patterned with tiny prints, the next it isn't and no sooner has the water receded then the crabs scuttle out again, a relentless race to see which story will stick.

'Can I get you a beer, Mum?'

'That would be lovely.'

I fetch two bottles and pour one for her. She watches me and comments as her glass begins to bead sweat, 'That looks nice and cold' she says, with a laugh.

I sit opposite her and raise my bottle before I sip, 'Cheers, Ma.'

At night, when the breeze drops, the ocean's song will seem louder and I will think of the conch shells my father held to my ear as a child: 'Can you hear the sea?' he'd ask and I would listen intently and then politely I would tell him that yes, yes I could. The rush of blood in my ears as a tidal hymn.

We are quiet for a bit then, Mum and I, drinking in the darkening view and our beers. Stars begin to puncture the sky with sputtering pinpricks of brightness. They appear, one after the other, as if some celestial body is putting a lit match to the wicks of overhead lamps.

And then, it was then, as the day sunk to its haunches, that Mum said: 'Tell me,' and she leant towards me, 'When did we first meet?'

⋆

Afterwards, I will understand better the watery metaphors that drench Dementia; when you start to look, to *listen*, you hear them everywhere: Dementia is described as a 'wave', a 'rising tide', an 'emergent tsunami'. Politicians, poets, academics wade through the language, sieving it for the right words. Dementia is flooding services.

But what I learn myself is that long before we, the well,

feel the cold rise of that tide, the sick have already begun to drown.

★

Later I will also understand that we all do what I did in the face of Dementia: make excuses.

She's overtired, I told myself when Mum could not follow a conversation, perhaps she needs a nap. She's distracted, dehydrated, hungry – did she eat lunch? – when she asked a question that was not anchored by context or common sense. She's just old, her humour misguided; when she warned my vegetarian daughter she shouldn't eat marmalade on her toast because the skins suspended in the jelly were made from animal hide. She's having a Senior Moment.

And much, much later, when I read Ritchie's words, I know he is right: Dementia is only silent because we are not listening.

It murmurs its way into the world. You need to keep an ear cocked to this thing. It could be there in the background. It could be.

Listen?

I am not sure if we do not hear it because our ears are full of sand. Or because we don't want to. Do we miss it because we cannot imagine a fine mind – not *her*! – shredded? Does fatalism render us deaf: *it'll happen to us all in the end.*

So we, *I*, looked instead, for palatable, passing, *friendly* reasons for the soft, slow fraying of a person's – of my *mother's* – cognition.

She's overtired. She's distracted, dehydrated, hungry – did she eat lunch? Perhaps she needs a nap? She's just old; she's having a Senior Moment.

When I track back, when I think about it now, my vision lit

by hindsight, my head inclined to Dementia's soft, slow tread, clues abound. Hansel and Gretel breadcrumbs which I either didn't want to see, or dismissed as nothing of consequence. So I stepped clean over them.

I rake my memory now as if looking for something precious – my daughter's charm bracelet, a 21st birthday gift which fell off her wrist as she ran on the beach and I imagined it gone forever. I had almost given up looking for it when suddenly there it was, winking at me, a curl of silver in the sand. It is only then, when I look, when I really look, that I remember another morning, a year – maybe more – before Mum forgot me.

That morning, as we sat over breakfast, I noticed Mum staring at something in the middle distance.

'What are you looking at, Ma?' I asked.

'That plant,' she motioned, gesturing towards the lemongrass in a pot, 'what can I see beneath its feathers?'

I frowned, puzzled: 'Leaves, Mum,' I said, 'you mean beneath its leaves.'

'Yes. Beneath its leaves,' Mum confirmed, unfazed.

Nobody else at the breakfast table seemed to notice, not my husband ploughing through bacon and eggs. Not my son, thumbing his phone.

'Feathers.' The wrong word, slid in with such exquisite subtlety it would have been easy to miss.

One word. What's one word, one ordinary word substituted for another ordinary word?

Feathers for leaves.

Dementia was whispering.

But now that I've noticed it, now that I see it writ large in our lives, it screams at me.

Shouts. *Insists*: a person is diagnosed with Dementia every three seconds.

★ ★ ★

There must have been a second split by disbelief.

Like when you've been slapped across the face: a moment before you feel the sting of it, seconds before the rose blooms on your cheek. A tiny lapse into which the shock drops before time catches up with you and you realise what a person has done.

Said.

'Tell me: when did we first meet?'

And then I laughed. I burst out laughing with such force, beer comes out of my nose and stings the back of my throat. She must be joking.

Do we all have a Before and After in life? A defining, separating moment?

A place where the seam of what came first and what came next shows? If we do, this is where mine came undone.

If your mother does not know you, who are you?

If she has forgotten her history, what's yours?

Before.

After.

'You've known me since the day I was born, Mum! You're my mother!'

(As if that word, *mum*, interjected by a lifetime of habit, were not enough of a clue.)

Her face blanches and her mouth falls open.

I can tell she is not joking. I can tell by the look on her face – her expression is hollowed by something like shock. I can tell by the tone of her voice; she enunciates a tight little, 'Oh,' in response to my laughter, my 'you're my mother.'

There is silence.

My own daughter, my youngest, Hattie, will tell me later:

'You went so pale, Mum.' I could feel the reassuring warmth of her hand at the base of my spine.

I need to say something to plug the breach that our story is already beginning to leak out of. But I don't know what to say. I've said it: I am who I am.

It is only months later that I will wonder: what would be worse, that your mother does not recognise you? Or that you do not know your own daughter?

I hope that by tomorrow this – this what? Confusion? Lapse? This transient, jarring Senior Moment – may have been forgotten. Or softened as something we might laugh about.

But it isn't.

As I step onto the hot veranda with a tray of tea, it is clear Mum has clung onto last evening's encounter and has been ruminating on it. She is pacing. She seems seized by a strange, alienating energy, as if lit up by some urgent underground current.

She does not look like my mother.

She launches in without using my name, 'Now. Now, listen, I've been awake all night worrying about this…' and she raises a hand to sift the air with her fingers, filtering it for the right word '…About all this *nonsense*, and I know you're wrong; I know you're telling me stories; you can't be my daughter. I know who my children are! I know!'

We stand facing one another in the full glare of the morning sun and one another's expressions. My mother is very close yet she feels very far away: as if she has wedged something sharp into the split seconds dug by Before and Afters, and wrenched us apart.

I feel a fretful finger pulling at a loose thread – the damage that can do in seconds! I feel that unravelling, a curious unspooling of time; I don't know it yet but the distance my mother will travel from me has only just begun.

'You are,' Mum states with assuredness, 'far too old to be my daughter.'

She sounds so certain, so resolute, so *confident.*

And briefly I am cast back twenty-five years to a memory of a quite different woman, a woman watered down by Depression to such timidity she told me, 'I think I need to go to lessons in assertiveness.' And I remember not being surprised that she needed to learn to assert herself – that much was clear – but that there was formal provision for this: classes in the art of saying 'No!'

'You must be at least fifty!' she spits, 'I am not old enough to have a daughter your age.'

Another memory – so many so suddenly – that I will wonder if they crop up coincidentally or reflexively, to test that my own recall is still functioning and accurate – this time, a photograph.

When my son, my first born, was just a few days old, I, 25, stood at the back door of Mum's Northamptonshire home with my baby swaddled against me. An unfamiliar shape in unpractised arms. The late summer afternoon has toasted the walls of the house so that they are caramel coloured, weeks of no rain and the lawn where the photographer stands is desiccated so that the grass is Africa-yellow. The brightness flares in the lens so the sun is caught in my hair, my cheeks flushed with the warmth. I am flanked, in the picture, by Mum who is fifty and my grandmother Alice, who is 75. What neat symmetry, we remarked to one another then, laughing with delighted self-satisfaction that we had achieved this clever balance. Each a tidy two and half decades apart. A generation apiece. Four collected on that back step that early September evening.

But there is no symmetry now, the maths is muddled, an abacus broken so that beads roll away where they cannot be collected or counted.

Whatever face Mum looked at in the bathroom mirror that morning was not, apparently, old enough to be the face of the mother of the woman she glares at now, with a mixture of suspicion and something else. Disgust?

I persist. I can make this add up, I can. I will.

I ask her, pleased I have thought to (for surely she will have no answer for my question other than the obvious): 'Why would I call you "Mum" if you weren't my mother?'

She shrugs. Her response is both instant and indifferent, she doesn't even need to think about it: 'Because you don't know what else to call me,' she sniffs.

Don't know what else to call me.

I feel Hattie's hand on my back again.

'I promise you, Gran,' she says, 'I *promise*, you're Mum's mum.' And she brandishes a trump card, ambushes her grandmother with persuasive logic: 'Otherwise how could you be my granny?'

Mum loves Hat. This thought stills her for a minute. She may be prepared to renounce me but Hat and her beautiful youth still make sense – she can believe Hat is her granddaughter. She *wants* to believe Hat is her granddaughter.

Later that day, frantic to provide proof of our relationship – you *really* hadn't heard Dementia's surf-roll before now? I hear you ask in some astonishment (No, no, truly I had not) – I scour my laptop for old photos. If I can only produce compelling evidence of my connection to my mother, I tell myself: some corroboration of my story, testament to the facts: See! You *are* my mother.

After

Much later photographs will be proof of nothing. They will simply be a portrait gallery of mostly unfamiliar people in a bound book. If my mother stumbles upon an image of her parents in those pages, she will remark with surprise, 'Oh look! Mum and Dad!.'

Her tone speaks of astonishment to find them here, her kin among those of this strange woman, as if to ask, 'What are *they* doing here?'

You imagine that because a camera can capture a moment in time, like amber embracing an insect, the profile of a particular occasion, or place, or person, will remain forever sharp and clear: you have pasted it to celluloid so that everything about that moment is suspended forever. A memory preserved in time even as time itself slides by.

But you are wrong.

'Who's *she*?' Mum asks one day much later as we leaf through albums. She is pointing to the young woman in the photograph with a bundle in her arms standing between her mother ('That's me,' says Mum) and her mother's mother, ('And my mum'), their backs against a stone wall toasted caramel in late summer sun which has baked the lawn in front of them Africa-yellow.

'I don't think I know her,' she decides. And she turns the page.

★

I find a slew of them – that afternoon – old photographs, in a folder on my laptop: My mother as a child in India, me at nine months on her lap, me beside my maternal grandmother. I collect all these pictures up and plant them in a PowerPoint as a family tree. I root myself firmly. A common denominator, branching out in connection to all Mum's people – her parents, her siblings, her husband – my father. If I can provide illustrative proof, I tell myself, I will endorse myself as her daughter, reassert myself in her affections, her trust, her *life*.

I show her later, when I am composed, when it's cooler, when I have bribed her to submission with another cold beer.

'Can I show you something…Mum?' I ask, my voice faltering; I am uncertain what I should call her in this hiatus of unknowingness.

She is reluctant at first. But curiosity gets the better of her and she sits down beside me, close enough to see the screen but not so close that our thighs touch.

A week ago, had I shown her pictures on a screen, she might have rested a hand on my leg, or draped an arm about my shoulders. Not now: now I feel the draught of distance.

I talk her through all the images I have collated.

'There we are with Dad – see – you, Dad, me?'

'There's you, Granny and Grandad – and me?'

'That's you and Rob and Carol – my brother and sister – and me.'

Later on, we will adopt this as a habitual trick, a subtle pointer to who's who; later on, we will learn to prefix a person's name with their connection to her or to one another: 'That's your son, my brother, Rob; that's Carol, my sister, your youngest daughter, with your husband, my – her – dad, Jim.' As if we are reinforcing the scaffolding of some ancient old building that's beginning to crumble and collapse.

And that's me, Mum, me, me. Me and you, Mum.

She studies the picture I am pointing at. I notice her eyes

slide to regard my face, 'Oh yes, I see, it is you!' I think I can hear relief in her tone. That she has placed me?

That I'm not lying after all? But I'm not sure.

For a few days after that, I hope Mum has recognised her mistake and recognises me.

But, it turns out, she has either forgotten who I am all over again or she is politely humouring me. Perhaps she was just trying to avoid another tedious who's-who-in-the-zoo PowerPoint as I tried to pitch myself into position of her daughter.

In the end, I think she is just waiting for back-up.

★

When my sister, Carol, arrives a week later to join us for Christmas, Mum aligns herself with her tightly, like a child might with the appearance of a more popular peer in the playground. And she begins to view me with growing and cold suspicion.

She takes a seat close to my sister at breakfast time, sitting as far away from me as possible so that she can scrutinise me, from the other side of the dining table. She squints at me over the top of her mug of tea, I can feel her stare upon me through steam.

Every evening, for weeks before my sister's arrival, I would accompany Mum to her bedroom, to turn down her bed, switch her lamp on, count her pills out into the palm of her hand.

Sometimes Mum asks, 'What are all these for?'

'These are to protect your heart, they're blood thinners,' I say, holding out the clopidogrel on the flat of my hand to show her, 'These are statins,' I say, 'they keep your arteries nice and clear. And these are Vitamin D, to keep your bones strong.' Mum smiles at me. 'And these,' I say, as I count out five more tablets, 'these are your antidepressants.'

Sometimes Mum picks the capsules off the palm of my hand, one by one, and swallows them with sips of water from the glass I hold out to her like an obedient child.

Sometimes she scoffs, 'Depression? I've never had anything like Depression!'

I say then, 'You did once, Mum, a long time ago.'

But with the arrival of an ally, there is a jarring shift in this evening routine.

When I motion it's time for bed, Mum insists Carol help. She holds out a hand to her, 'Come, come, please come,' she says in a voice enfeebled, I am appalled to notice, with something that sounds like fear.

When I rise too, and make a clumsy, confused attempt to insert myself into this cosy union, 'Let me help,' Mum shoots me a look: 'No, thank you' she says, 'I don't need you; she' – gesturing Carol – 'is here to help me. Goodnight.'

You. I don't need *you*.

She gives me a tight little smile and shuts the door in my face so that my toes are almost caught beneath it.

I stand on the other side of the closed door and lean my forehead against it. I can hear her chatting cheerfully to my sister who is silent because, I imagine, she is studying the pharmacist's unfamiliar scripts as she counts pills out. She will, I think, be checking them against the notes I wrote and which are kept with Mum's drugs. In case. In case what? In case I'm not there and somebody else must take charge.

I never imagined it might be for this reason.

⋆

Days later I slyly listen in to Mum on the phone to her own sister because, in my bid to understand this alienating development, I have taken to eavesdropping on her calls, on all her conversations.

'Apparently Anthea is my daughter!' she exclaims, 'I wish somebody had told me! Did you know?'

It's only months and months later that I recognise it's not just the lost memory that is troubling, not just the dimensions of that misplaced memory (how do you forget your *daughter*?) it's the way Mum tries to make sense of the forgetting, the way she places blame for this at somebody else's feet: *I wish somebody had told me.* If you thought Dementia was just about forgetting – and I did once – you are wrong. Forgetting is only the beginning. It's that first fretful finger at that loose thread. It's the skewed logic in trying to make sense of the forgetting that begins to pull the whole thing apart. My eldest daughter, Amelia, is appalled at her grandmother's unravelling.

'How does it make you feel, Mum?' she asks.

I don't know how I feel. How am I supposed to feel? Hurt? Angry? Confused? Should I be grieving? (Yes, I learn later: you should be grieving. Another metaphor: *Dementia is a living death*).

I feel hollow. I feel as if a huge part of my history has been torn out and ripped to pieces and set fire to. I feel as if my identity is a lie.

'I feel rudderless,' I tell her, 'Like I've lost my bearings.'

Mostly, though, I just feel sad: sad at the furtive, suspicious looks Mum gives me across the breakfast table, sad at her evident distrust of me. And sad that I begin to feel scared, scared of spending time alone with her, because the lack of trust stings and I don't want to have to defend my position again. Subtly the distance sliced that evening is split further and further apart, the widening chasms of seismic shift. We avoid one another.

Three weeks later, Mum leaves to return to a wintery Ireland. As I hug her goodbye, I feel her stiffen, just as you might if a stranger were to encroach on your space. I kiss her on her cheek. I scold her gently as I smile, 'Now, Mum, don't forget me.'

March 2020 (After)

Within weeks of my mother's return to Europe, the world is strait-jacketed by pandemic: she's locked down with my brother and his family in a rule-bound, mask-wearing, socially distanced corner of southwest Ireland and I'm in a flagrantly Covid-denying red-listed country in Africa where caution is thrown to a dusty wind and we are urged to put our faith in lemon, ginger and the gods. Churches are packed.

It will be more than a year before Mum and I see one another again.

I ask myself afterwards whether the Coronavirus-crusade I embarked on was an altruistic endeavour to keep my mother engaged during that peculiar isolating time when – as a woman in the at-risk over-seventy category – she wasn't even allowed to accompany my brother to the local supermarket.

Or was it a desperate last-ditch attempt to reinstate myself as her daughter? A sort of virtual inveigling as I attempted to wheedle my way back into her world?

The first time I speak to Mum on Skype after her return, I do so with some trepidation and my brother's support; it is clear he has primed her. I imagine him standing close and prompting her with cues, propping up that falling-down familial scaffolding.

She wishes me a belated Happy Birthday, 'I'm sorry I forgot it,' she says.

It's happened before. For another reason. Though I don't say that. I just say, 'That's okay, Mum.'

And then she says, 'And I'm sorry I didn't believe you were – *are* – my daughter; you must have been very hurt.'

It sounds almost comical. As if she were apologising for forgetting something trivial. As if this important connection had just slipped her mind. As if – in fact – she was apologising for having forgotten my birthday.

'That's okay, Mum.' Again.

* * *

Ironically, days after Mum enquired when she and I had first met, my siblings and I gave her an Echo Show, an Alexa device with a screen.

Voice-controlled, it meant she could summon us up with a single command:

'Alexa, call so-and-so.'

And Alexa would obediently Skype me or my sister or my aunt.

It worked well until Mum forgot Alexa's name and it became 'that bloody woman'.

And Alexa, who does not respond kindly to cursing, especially if you don't use its – her – name, did not respond at all.

Irony abounds when, despite Alexa's high definition eight inch display, Mum cannot see me.

I told my brother before that first call, 'I'm not going to put my camera on: I can't go through that again.' He knows what I mean.

So, Mum cannot see me, but I can see her: when she picks my calls up, I watch her face swim into my screen. Sometimes I see her bedhead, a towel slung over it. Sometimes I see the ceiling. Occasionally just the top of her head – so that I can tell – depending on whether her hair is brushed or not – how the day has begun.

I ask her to tip her device so I can see her smile.

'Why can't I see you?' she asks.

I tell her it's because I cannot turn my camera on because my bandwidth is too narrow.

Mum is accepting of this; she does not understand anything of the technical link that connects us.

She can't see me, but always recognises my voice: as soon as she hears me, she says, 'Oh hello, Anthea.'

'Who am I again?' I tease Mum before I hang up.

'You are Anthea,' she says, 'you are my daughter; you are *that* Anthea,' as if she has been rehearsing the characters of a cast.

That Anthea.

I call her every week during the pandemic, often daily. Some days our calls feel strong and tethering.

On others, our connection is tenuous: she is distracted or distressed and cannot get a grip of the conversation or who we are in relation to one another, or where we are. On those days it feels like a rope fraying.

On those days it feels as if the mooring of a small boat is being tugged by wind and tide and is in danger of being pulled right out to sea.

Chapter 2: Deep Blue

March 2023 (After)

I was once interviewed on a small radio show called *The D Word*, about Dementia.

The D Word. Like the F word. A word we don't want to say out loud, in full, for fear of inciting fear or insulting sensitivities.

Or tempting fate: if we don't say it, perhaps we won't summon it into being. As if in keeping the whole word contained in our mouths, and only whispering a clue, *The D Word*, we're touching wood (*Please. Not me.*)

The D Word. Is that all, I puzzled then, at the time: Just D for Dementia?

What about D for death?

When death overwhelmed us later, it took us by surprise: we didn't see it coming, didn't hear a thing, and when it came, it wiped out everything that had come before. Flattened us. Meant we had to wade chest-deep through its high cold waters and pick out what we could find from the detritus so we could cobble together some new version of our lives. We definitely never expected D for death.

And what about D for Depression?

That was different. Depression is not silent. I heard it; I knew something was coming. I just didn't know what.

★ ★ ★

I am sometimes struck that I could travel the distance between not knowing a thing about a condition, and needing to know absolutely everything about it once it caught my attention, in such a short space of time. I have since found that I am not alone. I speak to a friend whose mother shares my mother's diagnosis of Dementia.

'I never used to think about it,' she says, staring into her coffee, 'Now I can't think about anything else.'

And it's all we can think about for two reasons: we need explanations for the strange ways our mothers begin to behave; we are forced to rationalise behaviour that is no longer rational.

And we're terrified we'll end up like them.

I am conflicted by the peculiar sensation of needing to get as close to my mother's illness as I can to stay close to her. And at the same time, getting as far away from it as possible.

My arm's-length ignorance of Dementia was foreshortened when the illness was dragged horribly close and became personal. Oblivion mutates as obsession and I begin to seize on every news item about the illness, every new understanding of it. I struggle through academic reports with a forensic eye.

I have done this before. With Depression. To understand my mother then. And to avoid the same diagnosis myself.

1978 (Before)

At first, we did not know, did not guess, Mum was ill.

At first she just seemed distant. As if preoccupied. Or tired. As if she might be coming down with something.

I try to capture this unsettledness in my diary in the round, even hand of a twelve-year-old: 'Mum wasn't feeling too good this morning, so she went for a lie down.'

* * *

I have tried to understand often since. If I heard Depression slink its way into our lives, why didn't I hear Dementia coming? How come – at twelve – I could recognise something was wrong with Mum and four decades later, I failed?

How come, long before the phrase 'mental illness' was painted to our everyday lexicon with a broad brush so that every sadness and disappointment and twinge of anguish was whitewashed as illness even when it wasn't, how come I knew then something was amiss even if my mother's doctor couldn't put a name to it?

I have analysed this, turned the conundrum over and over in my head and think I understand why now.

As children, our faces are turned inwards, towards our parents. They are the centre and the sunshine and the nourishing force of growing lives.

*

When I was a child, food was a thing of happiness. Every meal was eaten at a table properly laid. Mum threw a linen cloth over a polished surface and leant low to smooth its creases with a flat hand. Cooking became central to my growing up. 'What shall we bake?' Mum asked, and we would pore over cookery books, elbows on kitchen counters, chins in palms, as we deliberated and salivated over the pictures in Katie Stewart's *Cooking Better All the Time*.

We baked in the afternoons, as if to nudge the day through its slowest hours. At my mother's side, standing on a stool, I learned to weigh ingredients, the tip of my tongue poking pinkly out of the corner of my mouth as I concentrated on the balance of the scales, old fashioned with weights described in ounces. Some of the smaller weights were missing, so we used a pile of coins instead.

I learned to artfully separate eggs and beat the whites with a fury until they stood up in snowy peaks, then Mum would turn the bowl upside down, laughing as I held my breath – properly beaten, the peaks would stay standing without slipping from the bowl.

I learned to handle pastry dough with a cool touch, running my wrists under a cold tap like Mum showed me. I learned how to whip a sponge to breathy submission; I beat sugar and butter and sunshine yolks to a cream of such velvety lightness that the air-filled batter seemed to sigh with pleasure.

We made Scotch pancakes and piled them steaming, swaddled in a clean tea towel. We ate them spread with Tate and Lyle's Golden Syrup. (Today, I cannot consider a tin of the stuff, lid sticky on my larder shelf, lion swarming with bees, without a sentimental swell.) We ate them to prove our half-Scottish heritage even as we grew up under hot, high African skies. I wondered, later, if that's why my maternal grandmother foisted Irish stew on us – to assert the other half of our Celtic makeup.

My grandmother's cookbooks were testimony to the cook she was. (She lived by the newspaper columnist Harriet Van Horne's maxim: 'Cooking is like love. It should be entered into with abandon or not at all.') The pages of her recipe books were glued together where flyaway mixture had escaped a beating, recipes had been altered in her own hand, a looping generous scrawl, others ripped from magazines and pasted inside the jacket cover so that the book was fattened on Gran's voracious appetite for cooking and collecting.

Sometimes – on special occasions – we baked a chocolate cake. Mum taught me to test it for readiness, the sponge pressed with a finger would bounce back to shape. Cooled, we filled it with buttercream; Mum cinched two halves together in a kiss-stained mocha with Camp Coffee Essence and we glazed it with icing spread to mirror sheen using a knife dipped in hot water. You could almost admire your reflection in it when we were done.

As children, we bask so close to parental warmth, hold our hands up to it, our gaze trained to a face so familiar, we are reassured just by its proximity, And when that closeness is splintered by sickness or when the light dimmed by Depression or the warmth replaced by a distancing coolness, it's as if somebody has turned a lamp low or a heater down: you feel the chill instantly. And when that parent loses their appetite – for food, for fun, for life – because it has been stolen by that clinical robber of joy, *anhedonia*, you notice the hunger everywhere. My siblings and I ate straight from the fridge then, foraging. Biscuit tins were disappointingly empty. Their shameful nakedness sheathed with a single stale sheet of baking parchment.

I, pre-teen, was so focused in, towards my mother, of course I noticed the infinitesimal changes as soon as they began to manifest.

Later, an adult, with the clamour of my own children, a husband, work, a life hewn separately from my mother, I was not attuned to her in the childlike way I had been then.

If you're watching the sea, standing staring at the place where it fingertip-touches the sky, you'll see the shift of the tide, you'll notice a sudden change in tempo and tug, you'll register the rise of a tide in a line on the sand, every wave draws it in again and again and again, higher and higher it comes, so that you have time to step back, keep your feet dry.

But if you are turned inland, facing away from watery horizons? You'll notice nothing then. Not until the water is lapping your ankles.

I had my back to her. How could I have noticed?

★ ★ ★

I was thirteen when a diagnosis was confirmed: *My mum has Depression*, I wrote in my diary. Just like that, with a capital D. Why the capital? Because Depression felt like a presence? Like a person. Because Depression, Dad said, is a Proper Illness? There we are: perhaps that explains my big D for Depression: proper noun, proper illness.

When Big-D-Dementia comes along later, it seems to confirm my capital D theory: these illnesses bring with them a personality of their own as they erase their host's.

I will wonder later if my mother's complicated relationship with Depression, complicated because nothing got rid of it for good, sometimes nothing got rid of it for long, was because of where we lived? Or because it was the Seventies? Or just because it took so long for Mum to receive a diagnosis that by the time she did, the black dog had sunk its teeth deep? It was never going to let go now.

1979

A long time afterwards Mum told me how the doctor had arrived at his diagnosis.

When the shadow of this mercurial thing that we could sense but could not pin down did not lift, Mum made an appointment to see her local physician. She sat opposite him in a small airless office and grappled with the amorphous shape of an illness which has no helpfully discerning physical characteristics. She tried to mould it with words that made it sound as bad as it felt.

She complained of tiredness, of aches, of not sleeping well at night, of not wanting to get up in the morning, of no appetite, of nausea, of an absence of interest in anything. Everything.

'Even my children,' she whispered, as if divulging some disgraceful secret.

Even my children. How strange, I will think later, that one illness left my mother ashamed she did not have the energy to acknowledge her children and the other without any memory of them.

Describing Depression is hard. It is like trying to describe an apparition; you can sense its presence everywhere but you can't see it, you can feel it but you can't touch it.

I am weightless yet I feel heavy, what am I?

How's anybody else to believe it's really there when Depression is a riddle?

The doctor listened, his brow furrowed. Then he took syringes full of blood. He tested Mum's iron levels; perhaps anaemia was the reason for her lassitude. It wasn't. He ran tests for ordinary illnesses like diabetes. Perhaps low glucose levels explained her lack of energy? Nope. Then he took more blood and tested it for exotic infections that may be lingering, for the ones that a childhood in Asia and a lifetime in Africa might have marked Mum with: malaria and brucella and bilharzia and tick-bite fever. He checked her heart, her blood pressure, her weight.

He pronounced her well. Except she was not.

Finally, Mum suggested, 'You don't think I could be suffering with Depression, do you?' She had stumbled upon a description of the condition in the *Oxford Dictionary*; she thought it sounded like the way she felt.

* * *

Let me just be clear here. My mother's Depression was not the 'designer disorder' a one-time president of the Royal College of Psychiatrists told me he feared mental illness was in danger of becoming on account of the hasty branding by prescriptions.

Hers was the train-wreck type, vitality-stealing, life-saturating, utterly, *utterly* alienating.

My sister will tell me years later, 'Even knowing other people now who suffer from Depression – they never seem to be as bad as Mum was.'

Depression, my mother's sort – recalcitrant, recurring, ruinous – is, I discover, when experience means I am forced to consider these things, a significant risk factor for Dementia.

*

A Danish study, one of the largest of its kind, followed 1.4 million Danish citizens, men and women, for more than forty years. It found that if you'd suffered with Depression in mid-life, like Mum, you were twice – perhaps even three times – as likely to suffer with Dementia later.

But why? Why might Depression in your thirties and forties pose a risk of Dementia in your seventies? What damage inflicted by melancholy then could erase your memories later? How could a visceral too-close connection with life ('Depressives are too in touch with the real world,' a doctor told me, 'That's part of their problem.') cause such an unhinging that my mother, in the end, seemed to inhabit some alternative universe?

Physiologically, Depression influences neurochemicals; it messes with the levels of things like serotonin, noradrenaline and dopamine. These drive changes in the brain. And the more frequent or deep or lengthy the episodes of Depression, the greater the risk for Dementia.

'On average,' I read, 'The rate of Dementia tends to increase 13 per cent with every episode of Depression.' *On average.* There was nothing 'average' about my mother's experience of Depression. Nothing.

A doctor will ask her years later how many episodes she's had in her life: 'Three? Four?' he poses.

Mum will look at him as if he's joking.

Mum's diagnosis – even if her GP couldn't put his finger on this lingering malady until she produced her *Oxford Dictionary* definition – morphed with time, and a pattern developed. Episode after episode after episode, each hard to shift no matter the pharmacological cocktail that was administered. Severe Recurring Treatment-Resistant Depression, a psychiatrist finally concluded.

Recurring.

'Reductions in hippocampal volume have been observed among individuals with recurrent Depression,' I read.

Hippocampus – from the Greek *híppos* for 'horse' and *kámpos*, 'sea monster' – those two small seahorse-shaped memory vaults that serve as a cache of our stories and a compass for our spatial awareness. Did Mum's Depressions shrink her hippocampi?

Recurrence of Depression in late life – and my mother's Depressions sustained into her seventies – cause 'subclinical cerebrovascular changes', as if the storms that howled in and out and in and out of Mum's mind eroded some elemental part of the brain's topography.

Mum's incessant worrying when unwell would have been fuel to the fire.

She tells me she feels afraid. 'Of what, Mum?' I ask, and I try to keep my tone even with no hint of the impatience I feel. It is hard to fathom what could hold such terror on a morning like this – a morning so bright it seems only to herald hopefulness – the sort of terror that keeps you curled in a chair, like a tight comma, a life in hiatus.

'I am afraid of what will happen next.'

It is that state of gnawing anxiety – 'rumination' in medical jargon – that causes the stress hormone cortisol to flow, then flow faster, so that it spills into the brain and swamps it, a body drowning in sulphur so that the eyes and ears and mouth and meat and bones of a person are dissolved and nothing of them remains.

And cortisol, Professor Ritchie told me, 'Can underpin the development of Alzheimer's Disease, by driving the production of the type of amyloid which lays the foundation for amyloid plaques' – the pathological marker for Alzheimer's.

He is at pains to emphasise two points: Some stress is good for us – it lends a sort of psychological endurance test to keep us limber. Secondly, significantly, these processes don't happen overnight. A handful of depressive episodes are unlikely to have a lasting impact on a brain. 'We're talking about "chronic exposure", months, years – for it takes years for the body's natural resilience to be overwhelmed – years of the brain being "steeped" in stress, just like it takes years of eating badly, years of sugar overload, to expose a person to the risk of Type 2 Diabetes.'

Chronically high cortisol levels are also associated with the loss of neurons in the brain, especially in the hippocampi. And so those seahorses, with their secret stash of precious memory and subtle skill in navigation, shrink some more. Mum forgot who I was. And then she forgot how to find her way to the bathroom.

Another study posits that there is a Dementia risk even if the first episode of Depression happened as long as twenty-five – possibly even forty – years before cognition begins to collapse like a sandy bank at a tide's rise.

Yet another finds a link between the number of episodes of Depression and the development of Dementia – is this the right word, 'development,' when Dementia by its very nature is a dismantling? – more episodes mean greater risk.

And Depression has a cumulative effect, as if the tiny slice of loose mortar – a first clue of a home falling apart – gathered momentum, became an avalanche of bricks until the whole thing collapsed, leaving Mum buried beneath the rubble.

I find Mum's experience of Depression in every paper I read, whether it was evident late in life or early; I find it in the recurrence of those episodes – every year, at least once a year, for more than three decades. I find it in the length of those episodes: the worst endured for almost two years.

Sometimes, I think what chance did she stand?

1979

For a week or two, Mum was consoled by her GP's words – you're exhausted, you just need some rest. She was reassured by the prescription for sleeping tablets that he wrote and ripped from a pad on his desk. She left his office buoyed by relief.

And who would not be encouraged by that? Who would not imagine that sleep was all that was required? 'If I could just sleep.' Aren't the burdens of whatever midnight anxieties pinch us awake in the small hours reduced to weightlessness by morning? Don't we rise at an acceptable seven and wonder why we were so worried at three, when all of the house was dark and still and blanketed by the muffling slumber of others so that you couldn't hear a thing except your loudly rattling thoughts? Isn't feverish nocturnal unease always soothed by the cold light of day, a cool hand on a febrile brow, when its menacing proportions are made smaller and we can see its shape clearly and realise with relief: 'Oh, it's not as bad as I thought'?

If we cannot drop back to sleep when we wake at three, do those monsters then loom large as life? Do they – with every sleepless night – grow bigger and bigger?

Mum's did.

As I grew better acquainted with the illness, I learned that this was Depression's habit, an early marker of its arrival and then its persistence. One bad night morphed into two. And then three. And then weeks of tossing and turning and tearful, reluctant risings.

Perhaps Mum's lack of sleep, night after night, week after week, month after month, snowballed into something devastating, something else that helped to crow-bar the opportunity for Dementia wide open?

(There must be reasons, I tell myself: there are always reasons).

⋆

We sleep in waves, our slumber alternates between deep and shallow-near-surface sleep when the slightest sound might jolt us wide awake. An onlooker can bear witness to where we are in our dreams by the flicker of our eyes behind closed lids in Rapid Eye Movement – REM – sleep. Sometimes, during this sleep stage, our fingers might twitch, our breathing quicken to mimic the faster beating of our hearts.

During REM sleep, our brain activity is high, similar to cerebral activity while we're awake, neurons flare faster and fire asynchronously. We dream more vividly during REM sleep.

But during Non-Rapid Eye Movement – NREM – sleep, those neurons fall in line as even, undulating slow waves. They fire simultaneously and tidily. We are more difficult to rouse during NREM, our bodies are slower, our blood pressure lower, our heat rate drops.

And it is during this deep, still sleep that our memories are played and replayed, and this results in a neural reorganisation that helps stabilise those memories, make them more permanent as if transcribing our day to a page with indelible ink. Scientists call this 'memory consolidation'.

An adult human brain weighs around three pounds, a tiny percentage of the average adult body. Yet it needs a quarter of the body's total energy to function. And in the consumption of that fuel, and in managing its smooth day-to-day operation, your thought-action-idea factory generates a huge amount of waste; every day, that adult brain eliminates a quarter of an ounce of worn-out proteins. In a year, the brain produces twice its weight in waste, waste it must dispose of in order to keep working properly.

And it is during NREM that the brain sets about doing this: its housekeeping chores don't just include the tidying up and archiving of our days, the filing away for later, but the cleaning up between those archives too. A job that's orchestrated by the body's glymphatic system which is virtually dormant while we're awake but hard at work during NREM sleep when the brain's levels of noradrenaline drop. This causes a widening of the spaces in the brain, so there's less resistance to the flow of cerebrospinal fluid which means it can move through the channels in the brain, rinsing them of waste, including toxic beta-amyloid and tau tangles, the signature stains of Alzheimer's Disease.

Neurologist Andrew Lees in his book about Alzheimer's, *The Silent Plague*, (that word again - Silent) calls this build-up of insoluble plaques and tau tangles a 'sepia galactic storm'.

I remember when I first heard the phrase – plaques and tangles; it struck me as almost poetic. I was in a hotel room, watching the news on television, overnighting between home and a flight. I was on my way to stay with Mum who had been looking after my youngest daughter for a month. When she still could. Look after another person. Look after *herself.*

I rolled the words around my mouth – amyloid plaques, tau tangles, amyloid plaques, tau tangles. As if in pinning them to memory, I was fastening a rabbit's foot to my collar to protect my own.

You never imagine, of course, that such phrases will become part of your everyday vernacular. That you will be forced to confront them, that they will lose all poetry then. Why, I asked Lees: why sepia galactic storms? What do they look like?'

Plaques, he told me, 'Are dense roundish clumps in the spaces between the nerve cells that contain the protein beta amyloid. Tangles are wispy, some are flame-shaped and contain the protein tau in a form which causes the fibres inside it to twist like a helix.'

And the sepia – which speaks to me of old photographs, of those captured recollections there, on the page see, secured by neat corners, fading to invisibility?

'Because the first stain used to clearly demarcate them was Congo Red which made the amyloid blush sepia.'

Lyricism of language is replaced by life-stealing facts; in my mind's eye, I see something knotty and violent and unstoppable, a tempest that roars through lives and turns them upside down.

And I think, is this some alternative amulet, this insistent asking of questions. If I ask enough, will I uncover the secret to saving myself?

2023 (After)

When I come across the phrase *anticholinergic*, I don't know how to say the word; I must revert to Google for instruction on pronunciation: *an.tee.ko.luh.nuh.juhk*, it prompts.

And I only come across it, long after my mother's memories have begun to abandon her, when a doctor I speak to remarks on the Dementia risk of sleeping tablets: 'Many sleep aids are anticholinergic,' he told me.

Anticholinergic because they disrupt a neurotransmitter – one of the most abundant in our nervous system – called acetylcholine – *uh.see.tuhl.kow.leen*, Google cues – which is essential for memory. It is, a researcher tells me, important in the conversion of short-term memories to long-term. Think of it as the programme essential to transfer data to a careful repository. The software to hardwire a past.

But acetylcholine has other roles in the body too; it's involved in involuntary muscle movement. It helps to regulate the heart and blood pressure. American pharmacologist,

Professor Reid Hunt, writing in the December 1906 copy of the *BMJ*, described acetylcholine as a powerful physiological depressor 'fully one times as active in causing a fall of blood-pressure as is adrenaline in causing a rise.'

If it was his intuition that told Professor Malaz Boustani, a geriatrician and neuroscientist at Indiana University, that these drugs may pose as insults to the brain, it was, he laughs, a scientist's necessary scepticism and research that bore his hunch out: anticholinergics aren't just bad for the brain, the burden of them is cumulative.

'The threshold for damage is between 180 days and three years of exposure,' he tells me. Just this one brief window in a whole lifetime, could be what 'tips you over to develop Dementia.'

And their weight adds up across different drugs; Boustani developed the ACB – anticholinergic cognitive burden – scale which registers a drug's value: zero means a medicine bears no anticholinergic effect, one represents possible anticholinergic effect, two and three represent a definite anticholinergic effect.

What about Mum's prescription, I wonder, what burden would that have brought to bear on her brain? And I begin to list drugs she has been on for years, adding a new line for each. I start with the earliest, old-fashioned tricyclic antidepressants, and the lithium she took for more than forty years.

I punch in: Imipramine. A red-for-danger three flashes.

And a message on the screen: Your patient has scored ≥3 and is therefore at a higher risk of confusion, falls and death. Please review their medications and, if possible, discuss this with the patient and/or relatives/carers. Please consider if any of these medications could be switched to a lower-risk alternative.

I type in Quetiapine, prescribed by my mother's psychiatrist years after another old-fashioned drug, Amitriptyline (three for danger), was switched out in favour of something else because, he had, he explained in an offhand tone, 'read something in the literature about it being helpful in the case of treatment-resistant Depression.' It wasn't. It made no difference; Mum's recurring Depression did not recede.

But Quetiapine loaded her score with another three points.

I keep adding, line after line: antidepressants, anti-anxiety meds, antacids (for even innocent, easily obtainable over the counter meds are not as benign as you might imagine).

Later, years after the anti-anxieties and antidepressants are prescribed, when Mum is in her seventies, they are joined by a medication for bladder control because acetylcholine is also the neurotransmitter that sends signals to your brain to trigger bladder contractions. If you suffer with an irritable bladder, an anticholinergic will block the message. My mother's GP stopped suggesting cranberry supplements when my mother didn't stop complaining about needing to pee.

The new drug scores another red-alert 3.

Aren't GPs aware of the threat anticholinergics (which Boustani tells me 'attribute 10 to 20 per cent of risk variants for Dementia') pose to the brain? Especially in the elderly, as more and more comorbidities present?

'No. Nope. Not at all,' Boustani says.

A clue that there's too little of this precious neurotransmitter in the brain might, I read as I scroll, present as 'Senior Moments'.

I squirm with uncomfortable recognition. Another symptom is the loss of spatial awareness (and I remember puzzling when my mother asked, again, 'Where's the loo?')

I wonder now if my mother ever questioned her doctors on the meds she was prescribed. If she had, would she have resisted the medication for her 'overactive bladder', if she had understood it may weight her already heavy drug burden with something that might tip the scales so her whole life was in danger of sliding into an abyss?

Even with the growing numbers associated with Dementia, I press Boustani, 'But with more and more people being diagnosed with Alzheimer's, surely…?' He knows what I'm going to ask. He doesn't wait for me to finish my question: 'There is zero awareness,' he tells me bluntly.

'But aren't there safer alternatives?' I ask.

'There are always safer alternatives,' he says, 'Always.'

That drug – that drug to quieten the pressing urgency to use the bathroom, which is prescribed to millions of elderly people every year – that drug added another three to Mum's score.

It brought her ACB tally to a shocking nine.

Boustani shakes his head, 'I'm really sorry about your mother.'

* * *

I asked Mum once, 'What's it like? Depression?'

'Like living behind glass,' she told me.

I think of Sylvia Plath's *Bell Jar*; she used the image to illustrate the suffocating nature of mental illness, a woman held hostage in the stifling sameness of stale air. When I think of the thick, cold walls of that jar, I think of entrapment, of the suspension of a life – 'I am inert,' Mum told me once – an atrophying exhibit in a museum; I can almost smell Plath's sour air.

Mum described it like this: 'You can see life but you can't feel it.'

You witness smiles. But you cannot comprehend their prompt.

You can hear laughter but you are deaf to joy. And trapped behind glass, a bumble bee incarcerated beneath an upturned tumbler, life didn't touch Mum; she was numb to her children when she was sick: our whining, our wants, even, especially, our excitement.

I thought about what Mum said often, I tried to feel something of her isolating position of silence and stillness and separation. I tried to place myself there, in her scuffed shoes and unbrushed hair, within her glass gaol. But I couldn't: my perspective – on the outside, on the *other* side – was quite different. From where I stood I could hear life rattle loudly: I could feel it as I was bumped and jostled and moved by its throng.

I can touch it and I am touched by it.

After

I do not need to ask my mother what Dementia is like. Years later, unprompted, she tells me anyway.

'I am in prison,' she announces.

I think it is the perfect metaphor for an illness that steals liberty, dignity and every single marker of a person's defining uniqueness.

But if Dementia is the jail my mother finds herself in now, I wonder if Depression didn't sentence her there when it robbed her of a life?

Neuroscientist Marian Diamond spent six decades studying the brain.

I watch her on screen now, animated, silver haired, her wide smile a crimson slash. She carries a hatbox onto a stage.

From inside it, pass-the-parcel style, she opens another box, then lifts out a Tupperware and then, from that, something veiled in a muslin wrap.

'When you see a lady with a hatbox,' she says, 'You never know what she's carrying.'

And from the muslin shroud, she lifts an adult human brain.

Her rapt audience, who laughed at the hatbox, gasp.

Diamond is famous for lots of things: those hatbox presentations; her YouTube lectures which garnered millions of views making her, I read, the second most popular college professor in the world; the fact that she dissected Einstein's brain and used an image of a slide as her computer's screensaver.

She rocked the scientific establishment when she posed that his brain contained more glial cells than the average man's and that glial cells were as important as brain cells and not, as had been supposed until then, some sort of secondary ugly-sister cells.

But she is most famous for her seminal work on rats. She observed that laboratory rats kept in cages with toys and companions did better than those housed alone and with nothing to amuse them. Her findings changed the way we understand the brain. Until then, the brain was thought to be a static organ, programmed from birth to follow a genetically programmed path. Diamond's work recognised that the brain changes throughout a lifetime.

'I looked at the anatomy,' she is quoted as saying of her lab-rat findings, the ones kept in cages with company and playthings, 'And found that the cerebral cortex – the outer layers of the brain – changed by 6 per cent. It was a difference between the enriched and the impoverished.'

Depression didn't just remap my mother's brain physically, make it susceptible to the inroads of Dementia later; the heist was broad and subtle, a peeling apart over years. It stole her appetite for everything, for fun, for *food*, so that for months she existed on an unhealthy diet of tea and biscuits. It kicked the legs out from under her, pinned her to a chair, kept her in bed, she didn't move for weeks. It hijacked her confidence and stripped her of self-esteem – socialising was an exercise in acute discomfort. So she stopped going out.

Diamond, who listed the five most important things for the brain as being – and in this order – diet, exercise, challenge, newness and love, concluded 'Take away the brain and you take away the person.'

If Depression robbed Mum of a life again and again, and it did, there was reprieve: she came back to us, again and again, her hollow shape filled in, her cheeks pinked, her eyes bright, her expression engaged and curious.

But Dementia?

Take away the brain and you take away the person.

Chapter 3: Rip Tide

Grief is consuming, like fire. A riptide that drags you out to sea. A vortex that tears you apart.

Carol Smith, *Crossing the River: Seven Stories That Saved My Life*

My husband, who spent hours free-diving beyond Kenya's south coast reef as a child, has an innate feel for the sea that I envy.

While I understand the superficial changing of the ocean's mood with weather – how it morphs from high hot day listlessness, as if even the tide doesn't have the energy for much except its soft rolling in and out, to wind-whipped waters that run with strings of wild white horses – my husband understands that what lies beneath its surface can be deceptive, even on calm days.

He says, of a new bay we swim in, 'Careful of the riptide, it'll pull you out to sea if you don't look out.' He has warned me often: 'Mind the sea, it can change in an instant. Appearances can be deceptive.'

I swim cautiously then, close to the shore, in the shallows, where my feet can still gain purchase on the soft sand beneath me and where I feel safe.

1985

A Monday in late June. I had woken with a hopeful surge that morning as clean, early summer light spilled into my room; the kind of feeling whose origin you can't identify, like sniffing the air for rain. Something was out there, something like change.

I had been living in London for four months. I was trying to make a new city fit as I tried to fit in, wiggling into a shape that felt very different, belts and boots and tight-fitting suits, jackets that restricted my movement so that it was hard to lift my arms to shoulder height, or raise them above my head, bare brown legs bound by tights. I wore a clutch of copper bangles about my wrist. Like a trademark. A childish signature of my Africanness. I still wear a tangle of bracelets. Silver now – the copper turned my skin green. My children tell me the sound of my clattering around the house reassures them; if they can hear my bangles, they tell me, they know I'm near. The same sound gives me away during a game of Marco Polo in a swimming pool, even with your eyes closed you can tell where I am if you follow the metallic jangle.

Even under water, my children can find me.

⋆ ⋆ ⋆

I am on reception duty at the office over lunch that day. The switchboard lights with a call. I pick the receiver up and announce myself formally.

'Hello,' says an uncertain voice, 'Anthea? Is that you?'

The voice, a far-away familiar voice which I'm surprised to hear – why's he calling? – is cleaved from me by time zones and distance so that the caller's words drag and slur and hiccup down the line.

Which is why the news came slowly. But not slowly enough. I would wish later that the gap in time had swallowed those words whole. So that it might never have happened.

'Your father's had a car accident.'

'Oh my God, is he okay?'

★

I left home for London on a high, hot night in February in the middle of an African summer, wearing too many layers in anticipation of my early-the-next-morning arrival in wintery England. I could feel perspiration tickle my sides.

My father is hopeless at farewells. Like me; tears brim just beneath the surface of all my goodbyes. We are similar in so many ways: the shape of our faces, the colour of our skins which turned toast in the sun, the same sun which bleached our brown hair blonder so that it looked like dirty straw. When I was young, people often remarked how much I looked like my father. Sometimes I wished I was more like my mother with her whip-thin frame and long neck and the deep hollows at her clavicles. She called them her salt and pepper pots, she hated them, but I coveted them; I curled my shoulders up and in to try to mimic the look as I considered the effect in her dressing-table mirror. Mum's skin did not tan so she stayed out of the sun; her creamy complexion never curdled. Her hair was so dark it was almost black and her eyes were a deep rich brown, like coffee, or chocolate, something sustaining. Mine were sometimes blue and sometimes sea green, turning on tides of emotion. Mum said they changed colour depending on how I was feeling. Or what I was wearing. I thought it strange, later, that Mum's eyes, with their constant colour, never gave her mood away. I felt as if they ought to have done: an early warning system.

I can still walk into a roomful of people, a roomful of people I have not seen for years, and they will still remark, the moment they see me, 'Gosh, you are so like your father.'

And I am glad.

*

'No. No, he's not. I'm so sorry. He's dead.'

I dropped the receiver so that it clattered to the desk. I slid to the floor.

Time stood still and time raced by and I spun in the vortex it whipped up all around me.

*

Afterwards, as I picked my way through the fallout, I would puzzle: shouldn't the phone have rung differently that day? Shouldn't there have been some hint at the news it would herald? 'Brace yourself.' But no, it rang anonymously, no name appeared as useful prompt on a screen back then, not the tiniest clue. It rang like every other call, a cheerful trilling to add to the chorus of ordinary office noises that day: the purr of printers, the sound of voices around the coffee machine, the occasional laugh, the scrape of chairs.

Later, somebody will toss the sandwich I had bought for lunch that day and abandoned after a single bite into the bin. Somebody else will push me into a seat and thrust a mug of sweet tea into my hands. I keep trying to rise, (To go where? To do what?) my colleagues kept pressing me gently back down: 'Sit, sit, drink, drink,' they urged. I keep lifting and lowering the mug. I agitate the watch on my wrist, twisting it and turning it against my skin, feeling the coolness of its metal, the slight heft of its silver chain.

Dad gave it to me as I left for London, 'For good luck,' he had said.

How much luck? Enough luck to turn back time? If I urgently rotate the hands anti-clockwise, can I direct those final fateful hours differently?

Later, later when I have time (time, time) to reflect, to gather up those scrambled hours and sift through them, I consider that at the precise moment of my father's death, I was sitting in an Italian restaurant on Battersea Rise dining al fresco. If I had made different plans, been some other place, could I have orchestrated a different outcome? At nine o'clock his time, he was gone. At seven o'clock mine, I was ordering a bowl of Pasta Puttanesca and a glass of Chianti. How?

'Where is your mother?' My kind colleagues ask, 'Was your mother with him?'

'No.' I shake my head, 'Mum is here.'

She had arrived two weeks earlier. I took the day off work to meet her at the airport. The moment I saw her among the milling throng in Heathrow's arrival hall, noisy with reunions, I knew that Depression had crept back in. I could tell by the way she walked – Depression evident in her slow, heavy tread so that she looked like she was wading thigh-deep through water. I could tell by the shape of her shoulders, bowed as if by an invisible weight.

'Sorry, love,' she said tearfully.

⋆

My father died long before so much of the inconceivable had morphed into the real: before the Berlin Wall came down, before the Soviet Union was carved up into today's component parts, and years and years before our world was spiderweb-connected by the whispers and songs and sounds that ring shrilly through the ether.

My mother used to say, 'No news is good news.' She used to say, 'Bad news travels fast.'

It travels faster now. Now it leaks out almost the moment it's spilled. Back then we could contain it. For just a bit. We could cup it tightly, briefly, in our palms as you cup hands to an ear to breathe a secret. Mark Zuckerberg was a year old the day my father died; we could keep our counsel; it was safe from Facebook, WhatsApp, Instagram.

My just-turned eighteen brother, mid-exams, was saved from the news for a week.

*

My father was cremated within days. His funeral was the first I ever attended; his coffin the first I ever stood beside. I watched it roll behind a curtain. I heard the roar of a furnace.

We bury his ashes with his parents, his brother, in the cemetery opposite the hospital where Mum had been treated with electroconvulsive therapy years before. I remember Dad pointing it out.

'That's where your grandparents are buried,' he'd said.

It's funny the places you know about but never imagine ending up in.

I began to dream about Dad soon after. And I continued to dream about him for years. Sometimes these unconscious meanderings brought me close to him – I heard his voice, could touch his arm, he is broken but here. There. Somewhere. In a rehabilitation facility in an unnamed place. They could not mend him, he explained, looking up awkwardly from his position in a bed, folded over injuries that were not clear to me. I woke on those nights grazed by optimism – *I saw Dad!* – until I came to, collected my tangled thoughts and remembered: he is dead.

Some nights, though, I woke to the screech of automobile brakes and somebody's screams and the sound of metal being sheared and there could be no doubt then: he is dead.

I told Mum, 'I dream about Dad a lot.'

She looked surprised. 'I wish I did,' she said. So I didn't tell her what my dreams were about.

Decades later, I asked a bereavement therapist, 'Why do I still have nightmares like this? What's the matter with me?'

'Your subconscious is trying to spin an ending,' he said, 'struggling to fashion something of substance from something that seemed surreal.' My father's death came suddenly, I was told over the phone, I never saw him again after the hot February night I left for London, not in life or death.

How was I supposed to believe what I had been told?

2005

Years afterwards, my children asked questions about a man they ought to have known but never did. I point out Dad's beautiful, unbroken face in photographs. He does not look old enough to be a grandfather, he does not look old enough to be my father, he looks younger than my children's father, life is upside down and back to front. As if the past has overtaken us. As if my father has yet to catch me up in years.

I feel a sudden spilling sorrow as I recall the day the picture was taken, I remember the occasion, I trace Dad's face in the frame. I read the letters he wrote to me when I moved to London. I stumble upon them while digging in a drawer for a pencil sharpener.

Can I really still smell his hand on the paper? Cigarette smoke and soap. The last was written a week before his death; he described his plans for an ill-fated weekend. I wished I could erase those words so that things might have been different. Strike through them with a pen. Rub them out and dust them from the page so that his plans were no more. Invisible. Unmade.

I ask Mum so many questions about him that she hands over the bundle of letters Dad wrote to her in the year before they married – a precious little collection tied with poignancy and a pink ribbon. I cried for a week after I read them.

Why? Why now – decades later? What was happening to me? The past had come back and prised me open and dug long cold fingers into my soul to pluck at it and pull from it things I did not know I knew or missed or grieved.

I am racked by sobs on the school run, so that my three children regard me with dismay.

'Why is Mum crying?' asks my youngest, perplexed.

'Because her dad's dead, silly,' hissed the older two.

They were too kind to scoff: 'Come on, Mum, he died years ago!'

Instead they gathered in a small huddle behind me, a show of solidarity and took turns to pat me on my shoulder as I drove, 'Poor mama,' they whisper, 'Poor mama.'

Feeling embarrassed, I speak to a counsellor.

Why now – decades later?

He tells me it is not uncommon to need to know a parent better as we become adults ourselves, as if we must find our feet in the paths our parents have worn.

Which is difficult if they are not there to share the routes they chose.

1985

We told ourselves: Africa will never be the same without Dad. Did we leave because we could not bear to watch the horizon from the veranda, the one we'd watched thousands of times before? Watching and waiting for Dad's dust: a tale-tell plume ribboning upwards to be frayed to nothing by the wind as he drove home: 'Maaaaaaaarm: Dad's nearly here, time for tea!'

What would we have looked out for?

And how could we have watched fat clouds, bellied with rain and promise, bruise the sky without seeing Dad bear witness to them, too, his chin resting on one hand, a cigarette in the other dropping ash carelessly onto the sill: 'Do you think it's going to rain today?' he'd ask nobody in particular.

We gave his faithful dog to friends, it was too hard to watch him moping about, his tail tucked miserably between his legs, his head bowed, wondering where Dad was to chuck a stick for him or whistle him up for a walk to the workshop.

He died soon after, of a broken heart, the vet said.

A long time later, of the same Africa, raw and jagged and wild, I tell my husband, 'If you die, I will leave this place. It will be too hard to be here without you.'

I think that's why we left: it was too hard to stay without Dad.

So we parcelled up boxes and memories and we left. And when we unpacked our crates in England, when we unwrapped the chipped, mismatched, familiar china that had crowded our breakfast table on the veranda, it looked sympathetically different in a Northamptonshire kitchen.

When we rearranged books on bookshelves naked of a dredging of African dust, they presented as a quite different library – except for the scent: when I opened the pages and breathed it in, the smell still spun from the paper as it always had. It still smelled of home.

When we propped photographs of the life we'd left behind up on the mantelpiece, we tried to avoid Dad's gaze: Dad always smiling, squinting into the sun, or laughing, head thrown back, a perennial cigarette clamped between fingers ('See if you can find a single picture of him without one,' Mum laughed as we arranged the frames.)

It wasn't just hard to see Dad's face in photographs because the missing hurt, it was hard to see Dad's face because it felt disloyal to be picking up and carrying on without him.

We saw Dad everywhere in Africa. But he had never been to England, so we saw him nowhere there. Except smiling from the mantle. It was easier not to miss him than it would have been had we stayed behind where his presence soaked every corner of our home, so wherever we looked we might imagine him: staring to the faraway line where heaven and earth met in a blur of dust or a blaze of heat, his hand held up to shade his eyes, 'Where's the bloody rain?'

No, we could not have stood to stay where Dad's invisible presence was so palpable – and as I write those words, I consider it is how I have described Depression a hundred times: unseen but tangible.

I am invisible but you can see me everywhere; what am I?

It was easier this way: to cast a new life in a shape that Dad did not fit.

We made a home in a small quintessentially English village. One with a red telephone box, a village shop with bubbled glass windows that sold sweets by the weight so that my young sister spent hours deliberating her choice, and a pub – Dad would have loved that.

I was glad he had never sat at its bar.

If all of this would have been alien to my father, who never lived in England, who'd never visited it, it was only slightly less alien to Mum.

'I used to work in London,' she sometimes told me: a tiny tailoring company in Mayfair, 'They made blouses.'

But that long-ago ethereal experience was brief and thin, as insubstantial as the silks and chiffons of the shirts they made. This one, this England now, was weighted with the baggage of children and responsibility and grief lugged by a widow too young.

My sister will puzzle, years later, 'How did she know what to do?'

Not just navigating a new life alone, but navigating a new life alone in a strange country: 'She'd never even shopped in a big supermarket,' my sister marvelled, 'Or dealt with heating. Or driven on a motorway.'

She had actually. Once. As a passenger in a date's car. A mile up the M1, she told me, 'When it was new, everybody was allowed to, an adventure, we drove with the roof down,' she smiled looking ahead, steady hands on the steering wheel as we carved our way up the same road, with the windows wound up to the whoosh of wheels and the roar of traffic.

Her grocery shopping had consisted of sending a list with a farm driver to the local store. They didn't always have what was on it. Sometimes she got surprising substitutes, sometimes nothing at all. She must have been a loyal customer: the proprietors gifted her a set of cheap saucepans one Christmas. She packed them up and unwrapped them in our new English kitchen, examining the enamel bottoms, 'These always catch and stick,' she said, 'They're not very good.' But we brought them with us anyway.

Now – like her new life – she had to navigate the aisles of new supermarkets too – enormous and disorientating, but mapped by numbers so you could find your way to the mayonnaise only to discover, when you found it, that you had to consider a dozen different varieties. In the farm store, it had been one. If you were lucky: 'Look at the choice,' Mum laughed, 'how marvellous!'

Six months after Dad died we celebrated a first Christmas with our first real Christmas tree, which shed green needles into the carpet so that Mum grumbled as she drove the vacuum over the rug time and time again trying to hoover them up, 'The sisal pole was a lot less messy.'

But we were wrong to leave when we did, as hastily as we did. We were not running towards a new life; we were running away from an old one. Within six weeks of Dad's death, we'd left Africa. You can't neatly pack up a life in six weeks. You leave bits and pieces of yourself all over the place.

We imagine that if we do not give a thing space in our heads, our hearts, it will not grow. We imagine if we keep it small and contained, we can prise it out, like a nut, the hard stone in the centre of a soft fruit, and discard it. We imagine that if we do not indulge the pain, it will never reveal itself. It will always be hidden deep within the softest part of us.

We should have given ourselves time, given death time to make itself – in dad's absence – felt, you have to pay grief heed, hear it, you cannot shove it out. Or set it aside. If you squeeze it into an ever-diminishing space, it will swell and press hard against every part of you until it cannot be contained and eventually it will come bursting out, messy, slippery as entrails, in illness or dreams or nightmares.

A year after Dad dies, another Depression unspools Mum. She falls apart in one of the supermarkets she has learned to find her way around.

My sister is trailing her with the trolley and rounds the end of a wide aisle to see Mum standing in the middle of it, weeping, her head in her hands.

'What's the matter, Mum?' she asks.

'The bread,' Mum cries, 'there's too much bread, I don't know which one to get.'

2019 (Before)

Mum is distraught when, years after dad dies, she loses her wedding band. She had lost her engagement ring decades before that. It had grown too tight around knuckles growing gnarly and arthritic so she wore it on her little finger.

'I'll get it resized soon,' she kept promising, but she never did and so one day it was there and the next it wasn't.

It's why we turn the house upside down when she loses her wedding ring, it seems especially important to find it now. Inside the band was an inscription in tiny neat lettering, 'Lala

Love Jim,' the gold thinning on the underside from fifty years of wear.

We hunt everywhere. We can't find it anywhere.

I can feel Mum's sadness, a sort of troubled dislocation, another important link broken. She wears no marker of her long union with Dad now.

She and my father were married in December 1964, in the promising hiatus between an old country and a new one, populations pregnant with anticipation; they married exactly one year after Kenya got its independence.

Mum was Irish from India, Dad Scottish from Kenya and here they were, a young couple in a young country with pockets full of newly minted coins bearing the profile of an African president instead of that of an English queen and a slim gold band placed upon a new bride's finger. They must have been so full of dreams and plans.

I watched Mum after her wedding band was lost, I watched her twisting the skin on her finger where it should have been, plucking at it. I watched worry at that loss cloud her face. But with time, she fretted less. She stopped asking, 'Has anybody seen my wedding ring?'

* * *

What happens when you spend years and years with the same person? So long that their presence shapes your internal maps so that when they die, you don't just have to navigate a new world outside, a world where they won't be – at your side, in your bed – but you need to keep resetting your internal compass to navigate around the spaces that were once full of a presence but are now wide with absence?

Research I find says that if you've been married for a

long time, especially if you've remained married in midlife, that union may bring some protection to bear on your brain.

The study, which analysed people between the ages of 44 and 68 over a period of 24 years, found that those who remained married throughout the period had the lowest incidence of Dementia.

Being married, say the scientists who published the study, means we are not alone in the face of life's stressors. We have somebody to share life's burden with, a partner as buffer.

Without that, coping with life alone might overwhelm us, might – given that unrelenting stress puts our brains at risk of the inflammatory stress hormone cortisol – be fuel to a kindling fire.

My mother was married to my father for 21 years. She was widowed at 44, missing those key years of companionship between her fourth and sixth decade which are known to be the vulnerable years when cognitive decline, if it's going to happen, begins to plot its path through a brain. She never remarried or shared her life with a significant other – for why should only those unions cast legally as 'marriage' be valuable?

★

Prairie voles mate for life. They are among just 3 per cent of mammal species that do. In a laboratory setting, a vole separated from its mate will struggle to reunite with it. In the wild, you might find two in the same trap, as the one will loyally, blindly follow the other towards a terrible end. If one of the pair is stressed, the other will demonstrate empathic behaviour, soothing with nearness and touch.

Scientists observing the cerebral responses of voles noted that the reward neurons in their brains lit up as an animal got close to its mate. The number of those neurons increased over time as the bond developed and deepened. The same thing happens in humans, it turns out: when we hold a partner's hand, the same area of our brain – the nucleus accumbens – lights up.

And that lifelong relationship between voles – because of the hormones that surge with closeness – changes their brains; the long-time presence of their mate is folded into the topography inside their heads, into the creases and pleats of their cerebellum.

My mother had to recalibrate her internal compass to navigate the spaces that were once full of Dad and left hollow and dark by his absence.

She had to navigate the coordinates of loss.

2022 (After)

One brittle winter's afternoon, many years after my father's death, Mum and I are walking around a small park in Ireland, the grass is spiked white with frost, the trees are skeletons against a bright, low sun. It's so cold that our breath leaves ghosts in the air. We have linked arms. Our nearness speaks to close conversation, our heads bowed toward one another, but in fact my arm though hers is more about guardianship; by now, my mother – her balance increasingly precarious – would be in danger of a fall without my support.

Emotionally, though, she is holding me at arm's length: I am not her daughter today. And because of that, she feels the need to explain something of the gaps in her life and I am always surprised at the detached tone of her voice then.

'My husband,' she says, in the formal voice of conversation she adopts now, 'he left me, you know; he just upped and left.'

★

A medic friend asked me once, 'Do you know how to tell the difference between a neurosis and a psychosis?'

'Depression is a neurosis and paranoia a psychosis?' I offered.

'Yes,' she pressed, 'but the difference between the two?'

'Go on,' I urged.

'The neurotics build castles in the air, the psychotics move into them,' she explained.

★

I, that day, that freezing cold day as Mum and I walked in a small park, was still poorly acquainted with Dementia. I didn't understand that building trust, a relationship, with someone who is losing their story means you must inhabit their disconnected world too, that you must conjure your own castles in the air. When Mum told me about my dad the deserter, I reacted hotly.

'Mum! He didn't. He died.'

Mum looks astonished: 'Did he?'

'Yes,' I say, 'He was killed in a car accident.'

'How do you know?' Mum wants to know.

'Because he was – is – was – my dad,' I say.

Mum is silent for a bit then, as she considers my words and her own careful step.

'Well,' she says after a while, 'Thank you for telling me that. I had no idea.'

My dad doesn't just die for her that day – or the day he died. He keeps dying because Mum keeps forgetting.

'My husband left me, you know,' she will attest, again and again.

'He didn't Mum. He died,' I tell her over and over.

It's only months later that I think to ask, 'Does it help Mum, to know he died, that he didn't walk out on you?'

I imagine my question is rhetorical, that I am doing her some kindness in revealing the true fact of this loss. I imagine that she will confirm, in response, 'Oh yes! Of course!'

But she doesn't. She considers my words for a bit and then she says, 'I'm not sure: If he'd left me, you see, he might come back.'

And so, before you know it, you're buying into the fiction of all this. You are living in some hinterland of make-believe, the Land of Let's Pretend. Before you know it, you are casting bricks from some intangible matter – helium or hydrogen or pixie dust, something fine as ash and light as a feather.

And in no time at all, I have moved into my own castle in the air.

2023 (After)

But as the weeks slide to months and as my mother's Alzheimer's claims more of her, as those sepia galactic storms gather and spread, my father is not mourned at all, not in death or desertion.

It is instead grief for her parents that mounts up and manifests in terrible ways.

This is the fact of my grandparents' deaths: my grandfather died more than two decades ago, from bowel cancer. My grandmother, whom Mum cared for at home after my grandfather's death, died fourteen months after him, following a stroke. Both were in their eighties.

This is the fiction of my mother's remembering, and

though the recounting of the story changes a little with every telling, the 'facts' as she recalls them remain largely the same: they always died within days of each other.

'Have I ever told you the story about my parents' death?' she will ask on a walk.

'I don't think so.' I always say because, by then, Dementia has stolen almost all of her past as well as her ability to focus on the present, so conversation, any conversation, no matter its provenance, is precious.

'Well, they went away on a hike/a safari/a cruise/a climb/a hunt' (as I say, the details change and sometimes the fiction is funny; a hunt!) and my dad got sick. He died very soon after he got home – within days – and Mummy, well Mummy was so broken-hearted she died just a few days later. Imagine. I lost both my parents within a couple of weeks of one another.' She looks devastated.

Sometimes I say, 'But they were quite old, Mum, perhaps it was their time to go?'

I say this because I hope the thought will comfort her, but it doesn't because she resists both the fact of their ages and her own: 'They weren't that old!' or 'I'm not nearly eighty! Nothing like it!'

Or she will argue the length of time that has lapsed since their deaths: 'It was NOT twenty years ago! It was only in the last year or so.'

So, I learn instead to say, 'I'm so sorry, Mum, that's a very sad story. That must have been very hard.'

'Yes,' she will say, 'It was.'

Sometimes then, to extend our conversation, she will enquire of me: 'Are your parents still alive?'

'My mum is,' I say. Nothing. No reaction. Not even a question as to where she is.

And, I add, 'But my dad died years ago, in a car accident.' There is not the tiniest flicker of recognition.

'Oh dear,' she says, 'So you'll understand how I feel.'

*

Sometimes, when my mother is especially distressed by the tortured, tangled world in which she finds herself lost, she will wail, 'I need my mother. I need my father. I need them. Why did they have to die?'

Salt into the wound of her forgetting. That big deep raw place that this illness has cut and cut and cut again in her life, dissecting all the good bits out.

And I will think – what other cruel disease does this: brings the long-ago loss of loved ones back into such sharp focus, even as it steals from you the loved ones who are still living?

* * *

A long time later, Mum's wedding ring is unearthed beneath her bed. It has tucked itself in a small nest of fluff and dust. My brother finds it as he lays waste to the debris that has collected under there with the Hoover.

We are elated, 'Look Mum, look! Your wedding band.'

She takes it between thumb and forefinger and considers it. She tips it to the light and slowly reads the inscription inside, before trying it for size:

'Who's Jim?' she asks

2022 (After)

When Mum has grown so frayed by Dementia there is almost nothing of her left, her wedding ring – and the coming and going recollections of my dead father – become peculiar anchors which on some days are tugged up and float adrift and on others remain securely rooted. I find this strange: that her memory of Dad is there one day and not the next.

'That's Jim,' She will say suddenly and with confidence as I push her wedding album in front of her, and again, on the next page, 'Oh there's Jim! Look at him. Always smiling. He made me so happy.'

But the next day, when I point him out in a photo and ask, 'Who's that?' of the groom whose arm she leans on, both of them slender and smiling and young, her hair a dark cloud.

She peers at the picture, 'I suppose it must be my husband,' she concludes, sounding a little bored as she turns the page.

2023

One day in the shower, many months after my mother comes to live with me, when she has grown so frail, so thin, her wedding band slips from her finger as I soap her.

She panics. 'My ring, my ring!' as it falls to the tiles with the tiniest ping.

I catch it before it vanishes down the drain.

'I've got it, Ma.'

'Oh thank God,' she says, close to tears, 'Keep it safe. Will you keep it safe?'

I dry it off later and bandage one part of its circumference in Elastoplast to fashion a slimmer band for much thinner fingers. I know to do this because she did it once to a too-big ring of mine.

Then I slip it back onto her finger.

'There we are,' I say, 'It won't come off now.'

'Oh thank you,' she says, 'Thank you.' And she holds out her hand to admire it, just as she might have done the day my father first put it on.

Chapter 4: The Octopus Mother

Nobody at the marina in Alaska where Aurora lived expected her to become a mother. She'd had an inauspicious start to life, found undersized, living inside an old tyre. She was four by the time she was introduced to a mate – old to breed in octopus terms. But shortly afterwards, Aurora began to necklace her tank with strings of eggs. Everybody waited, watching for them to hatch. But they didn't. They remained a pearly, sterile white. Assuming her eggs must be infertile, the aquarists at the centre began to drain Aurora's tank.

But Aurora, whose age showed in thinner skin and weakening suckers, refused to abandon her eggs. As the water levels fell, she desperately sent jets of spray over them cleaning them, keeping them hydrated and fending off sea cucumbers and starfish.

Daily, gallons of water were drained from her tank until one day, an intern spotted tiny, hopeful red eyes forming in the eggs and, to Aurora's relief, her tank was refilled.

She spent months more, then, devotedly tending her eggs, stroking them, wafting currents of water over them to aerate them, defending them from predators. She didn't leave them once. She didn't eat, the bit of her brain that had once instructed her to feed herself shut down so that all her energies were focused on rearing her young. She got smaller and smaller.

Aurora died as her eggs hatched as tiny quarter-inch-long replicas of their mother.

I relate this story to Anthony, my husband, 'Isn't that sad?' I say.

He shrugs, 'It is,' he agrees, 'but it's what mother octopuses do: they put everything into brooding the only clutch of young they'll have in their lives. And then they die.'

2017

That afternoon I had swum between tides, wearing a mask and snorkel, back and forth I drifted in clear-window warm waters, watching weeds wave beneath me and schools of tiny fish flit; the sea was strung with the smallest, smallest things which hung like dust motes might in sunshine.

That afternoon the sea seemed benign.

That evening was Amelia's last before returning to work in London. She was six hours away from departing. We were in the hiatus of goodbyes: simultaneously wishing them over and done with and hoping they'd never come.

'Come on, girls,' I said, 'one last swim.' To hurry time along or suspend it in distraction.

Hattie, Amelia and I headed to the beach.

The tide was low, the sea puddled in aquamarine and bottle green. We waded knee-deep then hunkered down so that our bodies were warm in soupy water. We talked and we laughed and we watched the quiet beach and wondered when we would be back. The sun was beginning to tip itself into the west and long shadows striped the sand like a zebra crossing. It would be cool enough to walk soon and afterwards we would open a bottle of wine, to drink to holidays and family and the New Year and then Amelia would leave.

We sat like that, rolling onto our backs from time to time, so that we could watch the sky, or we sifted sand at our feet to see what small treasures we might excavate: tiny, perfectly formed shells. We stayed there almost an hour and then I said, 'Time to get out, girls.'

We debated the best route back to the beach. In the event, we choose the worst. The water was still shallow so we crocodile-walked on our hands towards a path through the coral which bristled with urchins. We went slowly, sometimes resting on our haunches, feet planted on the sand, crouching low in the warm-bath water.

And suddenly Amelia said. 'Ow!'

And again: 'Ow!' And, then, more urgently. 'Ow, what is that?'

I thought, urchin? Or a toe stubbed on an unseen rock? I might have laughed at her expression, I thought she was playing. I raised her foot from the water to see. A puncture mark on her big toe was bleeding. Not profusely, but energetically. The blood ran in a thin river down her pale sole and back into the sea. And the pain began to build. And I thought: 'It is none of those things. It is not an urchin, it is not a stubbed toe.'

It is something worse.

Amelia had grown very pale.

I urged her out of the water; 'Let's get onto the beach,' I said trying to keep the panic out of my voice, 'Quickly.'

But the tide had turned and we were being buffeted by water rising. It was hard to keep my balance. Amelia cannot walk and she could not swim. She seemed disorientated by pain. Hat and I tried to support Amelia's weight through the water but she is taller than both of us and slippery with soapy saltiness.

'I can't,' she whispered, 'I can't walk.' We dragged her then, me by her feet, Hat supporting her head.

'Shall I get Dad?' Hat asked. She was beginning to look afraid. 'Yes,' I said, 'get Dad.' He was swimming not far away. Hat gesticulates madly. Waves. Wades through water fast and carelessly, mindless of urchins and rocks and coral and whatever it is that Amelia had trodden on.

Amelia's pain accelerates. She is beside herself now, breathless with agony. Her body arches back. It takes all my strength to hold this tall girl's face above the water, cradling her, telling her 'It will be okay, I'm getting help.'

I cannot make sense of what has happened. I only know there are no dangerous snakes in these seas. That's all I can think. What else can this be? I try to keep a hold of Amelia but it is hard in this quickening tide. Her body begins to convulse with muscle spasms. Her eyes are wide with fear. I tell her over and over, 'It'll be okay, it'll be okay.'

I don't know if it will be. I drag my daughter to the beach where waves meet the sand in mock-gentle caress.

A holiday maker, noticing our distress, rushes towards us; he is a doctor. He feels Amelia's pulse, 'Fast,' he says. I see a flicker of concern trip across his expression.

Anthony is with us now. He knows instantly that this is serious. He runs for the car, and brings it as close as he can. I hold Amelia tight, 'What is it, Mama? Why won't the pain stop, Mama? What is it, Mama?' I don't know. I can't answer any of her questions.

For a single awful second I wonder, will I lose my precious daughter in this beautiful place, a place my children love, a place their father, grandmother, once called home? I will hate it forever if I lose my girl here.

Then people are helping us to lift Amelia, four men carry

her to the car, writhing and crying in pain. I run up the beach, slowed by sand and panic so that my chest is too tight for air. My tongue has stuck to the roof of my mouth. I throw a pair of shorts and a shirt over my wet costume, I grab a towel for Amelia and then we are in the car, she, Ant and I, speeding to hospital. Recklessly. Ant weaves through tuk-tuks and drives vehicles off the road.

Normally I'd reprimand: 'Ant! Slow down.' Now I will him on: 'Faster, faster.'

I hold Amelia tight all the way, all 20 minutes of it. She is hysterical with pain now. I beg her to breathe. She throws her head forward and then throws it back. Her eyes roll up and I shake her and plead, 'Breathe Melie, breathe.' And I say it over and over and over again: Breathe Melie, breathe.

When we get to the hospital she is bundled into a wheelchair, in her bikini, a towel around her waist, a t-shirt thrown over her head. We are surrounded by worried faces, a doctor, two, and Amelia continues to beg, 'Make it stop, please, please make the pain stop.'

They inject lidocaine into her foot, briefly there is respite and I see relief flood her face. And then it's back, whatever appalling agony this is, it's back in a matter of short minutes.

Morphine. Pethidine. Nothing works. Finally, the attending doctors haul in the anaesthetist who tries to establish from my daughter, strung with agony, 'Where does it hurt? Where does the pain stop?' She motions to the top of her leg – the pain is climbing, her thigh is beginning to throb – and they draw a line with a pen at the place where the pain stops and then they puncture the line with shots of nerve blocker and finally, *finally*, there is reprieve. She can breathe.

A stonefish, they pronounce later: 'Definitely a stonefish.' There, in her big toe, the tell-tale black puncture mark is clearly visible, a half-moon bruise. IV lines are strung up about her bed, cortisone, pain relief and antibiotics flood her system to combat the venom.

Stonefish are the most poisonous fish in the world. They lie in wait, sluggish and ugly, like some monstrous, prehistoric species. They wear a camouflaged coat of armour, their small mean eyes are set deep in bony sockets. At the first sign of threat, they raise their dorsal fin as a lethal fan, threaded with 13 spines, like hypodermic needles, and inject their venom deep. Once, years before Amelia's experience, Ant caught a stonefish and laid it – still alive, for they can live for 24 hours out of water – on the kitchen counter. He pressed the end of a long cane into its back: the poison it expressed hit the ceiling. Fishermen nickname it the King of Pain and have attempted to amputate their own limbs to escape the agony; people have drowned because the pain has hobbled them, filled them with panic so they are disorientated and can neither stay afloat nor swim.

I used to imagine this pain was writ large by myth and legend, that stories of the agony stonefish inflicted had grown with their telling. Until I witnessed it in my daughter: Amelia would have drowned had Hat and I not been with her to drag her from that evening's rising tide. It is hard to write those words: my healthy, young, strong-swimming daughter would have drowned in two feet of water.

The pain is under control but the next day a fever builds and the swelling begins and Amelia's foot loses its elegant shape and wears a hot red sock of growing infection. By evening, the sock is pulled higher and her skin is flushed sunburn-red by a rising temperature. A second antibiotic is introduced. Marine injuries grow dangerous bacteria fast. I watch the nurses like hawks. I photograph my daughter's foot every day, twice a day, scrutinising the images for signs of change. I gaze at her pale face as she sleeps, her long dark hair fanned out, and I cannot bear to think about what might have happened had we not been with her in the water.

She lies in her hospital bed for five days. I spend hours of each of those days lurking nearby so that Anthony must insist in irritated tones, 'If you don't get out of here to eat or sleep, you're not going to be any good to anybody.' I track the medics who come and go and change drugs and then IV lines as her veins become resistant and inflamed with medication and toxins and fever and her own distress. She is pitted with puncture marks, blue with bruises. And all the while Amelia's foot swells. Somebody mentions gangrene. I talk to specialists at the big city hospital in the capital, to understand the best drug regime to contain this mounting infection.

★ ★ ★

A long time ago, when I first became a mother, there was resentment at my stolen self, an abandoned career and a social life surrendered in exchange for nappies and broken nights and the isolation and mind-numbing boredom that often attends early parenthood.

In the beginning, I minded that my identity had morphed from 'marketing' to 'mother': 'Just a mum,' I admitted – a bit bashfully – when asked, 'So. What do you do?' I hated that people seemed not to see me beyond – behind? – my baby, his father. I felt as if I'd receded into some sort of blurred background and had lost the sharp profiles of the shape I'd once inhabited.

Sometimes I felt as if I were disappearing.

My mother professed not to understand my disgruntlement, why being a mother, *just a mum,* just like her, wasn't enough. She scolded me: 'Know how lucky you are. Be happy,' she tutted as she held my tiny son up against her shoulder and soothed him with soft sounds and a deft handling that I hadn't yet mastered.

The paradox of my mother's assertions only occur to me now: she often wasn't happy. Despite her children. But I don't believe it was being a mother that made her unhappy. I think it was the relinquishing of herself to motherhood and then, necessarily, relinquishing some elemental, immersive parts of that role as we got older.

I asked her once what caused her Depression. She didn't have to think about it: 'Loss,' she said, 'your sister started at nursery; your brother went away to boarding school: loss. See?'

★

One baby became two and then three, so soon I had a trio under five and my shape changed again. The angular one on which city suits once hung softened and I grew curves in precisely the right places: my hips could bear the weight of a toddler; my sides could support my children as they curled into me when I told them bedtime stories. My lap was ample enough to hold a third there and still read a book to all three. Later, and for the briefest period – before they all grew taller than me – the hollow between my jawline and shoulder was the perfect place for a sad or tired teen to rest their head.

And my internal topography changed too: my children steeped my subconscious, tripped through my dreams, dictated the direction of my day from school runs to teeth brushing, from lunch boxes to homework, from class outings to Christmas holidays. Even when your children aren't there, a friend once observed, they're in your head, as you worry whether they took their PE kit to school or why they seemed subdued at breakfast or how the bloody hell they managed to get nits again.

But children grow up and leave your side – the side they've moulded to fit themselves snugly into. And it's up to you then to make sure there's enough left of you to change shape again, to close over holes and gaps. To fill in the loss.

2008

In the days before my son left home for London at seventeen, I wrote lists of all the things he needed to do when and where and how; relinquishing control when you've held small hands across busy streets is easier said than done. My mother still reached for mine crossing a road when I was in my thirties.

My eldest daughter witnessed my fussing and laughed, 'Do you know what Mum did the first time I went to Gran's on my own? She sent me directions of which trains to get and where to get off, and she wrote in big letters, **WHEN YOU GET OFF, REMEMBER TO MIND THE GAP BETWEEN THE TRAIN AND THE PLATFORM**.'

My children howled with laughter.

'Did I really?' I asked, feeling silly.

It sustained itself, that joke, for years: Every time I asked one of my children as they readied themselves for any departure, 'Have you got your phones/passport/ticket/bank card?' they'd chorus, 'Yes Ma! And don't forget to mind the gap…'

And when they left, I waved them off. And I plastered on a big smile to pretend I was as excited about their adventures as they were.

And I stepped back, then, into my emptied life and heard the silence and filled a washing machine with bedlinen still perfumed with the heady scent of children, gazed into a fridge that still bore the leftovers of last meals.

And I remembered that it was me who must Mind the Gap.

★ ★ ★

Bearing children, the research says, is good for women's brains.

Scientists at the University of California studied 15,000 women who were between 40 and 55 years old in the Sixties and Seventies.

Those who had three or more children were 12 per cent less likely to develop Dementia decades later, they found.

It's all explained by hormones, the scientists say.

Women are twice as likely as men to succumb to Dementia. (They are also twice as likely to suffer with Depression – you have to wonder at the connection). We live longer; age pushes the window wide open for this thing to climb in. But with age something else happens, a woman's neuro-protective oestrogen levels – which are at their highest during the third trimester of a pregnancy – drop off.

The loss of oestrogen is believed to lead to an increase in the production of Alzheimer's disease-driving amyloid, partly because women's brains are strung with oestrogen receptors. With a dwindling supply, there's nothing to switch those receptors on, they lie unlit in the dark, like tiny blackened bulbs of blown-useless Christmas tree lights.

I find a striking MRI image that shows a woman's brain before and after menopause. Before, the lobes are bright with activity. Afterwards? Afterwards they are dull, activity drops off by 30 per cent.

★

A study I read states the obvious, 'The transition to motherhood is associated with extraordinary physiological and behavioural changes.'

During pregnancy, a woman will experience unprecedented transformation – not just in the evident physical shape of her, but in dramatic fluctuations, not only where you'd expect – in the levels of circulating hormones – but also in cardiac response, blood volume, which increases by half again, renal, respiratory and immune adaptations.

The swell of abdomen as the foetus grows – from poppy seed to sesame seed, then lentil and chickpea – barely shows at first. I was fascinated by the pictorial representations I found as reference to what was happening in my body when my own flat tummy gave no hint of its hidden secret, first as grape, olive, lime, then revealing my condition as it rounded through apple and pomegranate to balloon as eggplant, coconut then melon.

Every day, nearly 400,000 babies are born. Their mothers, for the preceding nine months, have undergone this metamorphosis, slowly at first until the baby they carry affects profile, posture, gait. Such a common thing: to bear a child. And yet so unique: humans will only ever experience the tidal transformation swept in on that great wave of hormones during a pregnancy. And women achieve it every day as they surrender every part of their anatomy, first in the nourishing of the unborn and then in the delivery and nurturing of a baby.

And a body subjected to such seismic change means, of course, that the brain is affected, too: total brain volume shrinks during pregnancy and then recovers postpartum. Is this the pathological marker of the trauma left after each pregnancy, is that why some scientists believe women who bear five babies or more might be at greater risk of Alzheimer's?

So closely aligned is this business of bearing babies and the brain that even the gender of the baby a woman carries impacts her cognition: I smile when I read those women who are carrying sons have better spatial ability than women carrying daughters. Could there be any truth then in the old cliché that men are better at map reading?

★

Mum had her three children. (Not more than five, three). I give her a protective tick against Dementia. And then she breastfed them, *us*. Scientists at Cambridge believe breastfeeding might help to extend the protection bestowed by pregnancy on a mother's brain. One hypothesis posed is that this could be because breastfeeding stems the production of progesterone which desensitizes oestrogen receptors, turns those lights down lower.

Tick again.

And yet, and yet: my aunt – so near my mother in age they could be Irish twins, so close to her that Mum never forgets her name – did not have children. I spent time with her soon after her 81st birthday. I watched her and wondered at the difference. She could have been twenty years my mother's junior. Her intellect remains tightly wound. No evidence of the insistently plucking finger of Dementia that undid my mother. Why, I wonder: Why? Because she worked? Because she walked? Still walks? And fast. She laces up her sensible shoes and strides to the shops where others take the bus. Onlookers observe: 'Doesn't she move quickly!'

I think about the science of Dementia, and the answers the doctors are looking for. Needles in haystacks? So they are tempted to clutch at straws? My aunt who never married, who has no children, still has all her memories.

So, do the babies we bear protect us from some unseen cerebral blow which is not felt for years? Or do they inflict invisible damage in their passage in and out of our bodies and the turning up and turning down of hormones and stress and sleep?

Or is our Dementia risk elevated because in our lived experience as women, mothers or not, our brains are impacted more than men's, not just because of the extraordinary feat of our physiology but also because of cultural and societal expectations and change? Some of the science suggests that the evolution of the female role in the last one hundred years may play a part in memory decline. Research has found women who participated in paid labour between early adulthood and middle age experienced slower memory decline in later life, for lots of reasons: the intellectual stretch of occupation, the social engagement it delivers, the filling of gaps and the reshaping of roles when your children grow up.

Is that why my mother suffered later?

Mothers who didn't work suffered a memory decline 61 per cent faster over a decade compared to mothers who were in paid employment.

I watch a video where this news is delivered to a panel of women. Many begin to bristle and the show's host quickly, sounding a little rattled, explains: this is not about which group of mothers is doing the hardest job, or the best one. This is about how paid work might be better for a woman's brain, she says: 'It opens up all sorts of different pathways separate from the well-trodden one a woman walks at home.'

And I think: yes, because the more routes there are to a place, the less likely you'll get stuck on the only one you know when there's a roadblock.

I think Mum's Depressions evolved as frequent and relentless because she never fashioned draught excluders to plug those gaps, keep Depression's cold chill out. She never stopped up the loss when we went to school; her days yawned wide and empty.

And later, I think, it was into those same gaps and redundant nooks that Alzheimer's took root like an eager, insidious weed.

★

There is, in Africa, an ugly parasitic plant called Cuscuta which threatens entire ecosystems because of its rapid spread of attack. Its tiny seeds germinate and thread a scrawny root meanly in thin soil to anchor a skinny seedling, then the plant begins to grow – greedily – in the direction of a host. When it finds it – a spreading acacia that gives generously of its shade, a lime tree jewelled citrine, a magnificent bougainvillaea flushed with deep red blossom – it climbs fast and furious, fed on light and air and the stolen health of its host. It possesses scales – like a snake – for leaves, and as it coils long nicotine-stained strings around the tree, the acacia's canopy start to sag or the lime tree drops hard, dry fruit or the bougainvillaea begins to bleed dead flowers all over the dust.

Cuscuta is a canny and overwhelming guest – its malice is told in folk names: devil's guts; strangle-weed; witch's hair. It proliferates as a sticky, neon tangle across treetops; it doesn't kill its host too fast – not until it's found somewhere else to move onto. Instead it smothers it, suffocates it, weakens it, so that it is reduced to a shadow of what it was, so that it loses all its glossy green vibrancy and colour, so that it becomes jaundiced and vulnerable to a slew of other sicknesses. If Cuscuta doesn't get it, something else will anyway.

Alzheimer's disease isn't always cited as cause of demise on a sufferer's death certificate. Even when that's what compromised them to the point of end: weakened a person so that they cannot swallow, so that they become dehydrated and thin. So they cannot walk or move and begin to drown as their lungs fill with pneumonia and their blood grows thick with clots.

2022 (After)

Why do people say Dementia is a regression to childhood?

Why do they comment, 'Looking after your mother must be like looking after a baby.'

It's not.

It is nothing like that.

Babies reach and stretch and grow and seek out your face and smile. They are plump with curiosity and finding. Their smell is delicious, new puppies, tiny kittens. Their expressions are open and wide-eyed. They are always on the tip of tears or about to bubble over with laughter. Their bodies are full of coil-spring ambition to move, move, move, leaning plump torsos towards a thing: bum-shuffling and crawling and dragging themselves up on a table or the seat of a chair to stagger to a mother's applause as they totter across a room like little drunks. If they fall to the floor before they reach the outstretched arms of adoring parents, they seem to bounce. The falling is a part of the getting up and getting going.

My mother? My mother is none of these things. She is curled and crooked and broken. We never encourage independence, (we are her gaolers), never urge her to walk on her own, falls could be catastrophic. I lift all the rugs from her room. I regularly inspect the soles of her shoes for slipperiness.

The evolution of child to carer, mothered to minder, is subtle to start with.

I have used the language I use with my mother with my children. I will use it one day with my grandchildren:

'Do you need a wee?'

'Shall I help you brush your teeth?'

'Here, let me help you with that,' as I pull up a zip or buckle a belt.

It is subtle to start with. And then it's shocking.

A child will insist on doing up their own coat, their small fingers bat yours away.

Let me do it, Mama!

You must exercise patience as they tie shoelaces misquoting whatever Bunny Ears mantra you may have used to teach them.

My mother, on the other hand, at the other end of this care-giving, care-receiving arc, stands resigned and mute waiting for me to button her up or fasten her in.

The experts say, 'Let them do it themselves, extend the autonomy.'

There's a point to that in children, your patience a necessary part of their learning. It will get them somewhere: telling the time, tying shoelaces, dressing themselves.

But with a parent who is unlearning everything they ever knew? It'll get them nowhere and you will only be impeded in your day. Their reliance on you is a gathering weight. And time is tight. If I show her – 'Here Mum, like this (*remember*),' I will need to show her again tomorrow. And the next day. And the day after that. As if rolling Blu-Tack between thumb and forefinger over and over until it's warm enough to stick. It is relentless.

And it is shocking when my mother, all her poise and intellect gone, throws a tantrum like a toddler.

It might begin with the soft tutting. a clucking of her tongue.

'Are you okay, Mum?'

'Yes, yes,' she calls cheerfully from behind where I am working: 'I am fine.'

But she is not. The clicks get louder, the tuts more insistent. Her harrumphing grows more irritating and more distracting.

'Mum!' I stalk across the room to where she is tossing about in a chair, 'I can't work with your complaining,' I say, 'What do you need, what can I get you?'

Tea will help. Or a biscuit. And, yes please, another cushion here. And one there. She revels in the attention.

I accommodate all this and still it is not enough. My entire afternoon is slipping into one of wasted hours.

I get up again to tend to her.

'Can you push my footstool a bit closer?'

I do.

'Right. Can I get back to work now?'

She smiles sweetly, 'You can.'

Not five minutes later, she has started up again. I try to ignore her but when I turn around again to check, she is slumped on the floor. She has slid the length of the chair and across the footstool to land in a heap on the rug.

When I attempt to lift her, to encourage her to her feet, she cries out as if I am inflicting some great injury upon her, and I have to concentrate to keep my voice in check, to keep the tone and volume even.

Having finally reinstalled her in her chair, I drag the footstool a short distance away, to allow the space to stand, to exit. She shrieks, 'Leave it there, leave it there, I want it there,' and immediately all I can think about is my children when they were three: furious, unreasonable, unable to articulate themselves, flexing their will over mine. She is not childlike, she is childish. I feel a searing conflict of wanting to help and wanting to scream.

★

The other similarity between my mother now and my babies then? The nappies, though not the changing of them. Just the fact of always needing to have them to hand: cartons of them, purchased wholesale and banked under beds. Ready.

And the food throwing. Though the reasons for this are different.

A toddler would toss a spoon of cereal to the floor to test my reaction, to observe the speed of its descent, to giggle when the greedy dog snaffles it up. A toddler throws food as part of an experiment in life.

My mother does this to get rid of food she doesn't want. She has lost the imagination to hide it, which she used to do with great cunning – sandwiches, sausages, stews – so that I might find a trail of ants excavating a biscuit in her toilet bag, a sandwich wrapped between tissues like a little gift and stashed in a pocket.

'That was delicious,' she beamed once of a chicken casserole as she presented an empty plate.

'Would you like some more, Mum?'

'Oh no, I'm full up.'

By the time I found what was left of it, scraped from her plate and into a plastic pot and tucked beneath a pile of towels in her bathroom, the lid was bellied and about to blow itself off; the chicken inside wore a rank fur coat of mould and stink.

But as Dementia gallops on, snatching and grabbing bits of her brain as it goes, she loses the creativity to secret food away. Instead she just drops it, or tips her spoon upside down, no matter who is watching.

Weetabix is caked to the leg of a chair. I find the dog gnawing it off.

And a baby's eyes are wide and wanting: 'What is this world, what's happening out there, can I see, can I get there? What can I hear?' Twisting in a highchair, eager to get out. They are amused by Shaun the Sheep on the telly briefly, until a butterfly seizes their attention, or the antics of an animal, or the sound of the washing machine, or an older sibling's toy. Always, always looking for the next thing, leaning into all the new things, learning.

My mother's eyes are often glassy. Sometimes I imagine I can see an inner skin forming over them, like the third lid of a bird, which needs this peculiar piece of supplementary anatomy as protection for the speed of lives spent on the wing and on the hunt. My mother's life speaks to a stilling.

My children changed so fast when they were little: like small plants, nourished, they grew towards the light of the world. Fast. Faster than I'd have liked. If only I could have captured moments of that speeding childhood in a snow globe to cup in my hands for a little longer, to slow it, to take my time to look into so that I could look back. If only I could have distilled those first years as scent to dab on my wrists, inhale and remember.

No. Looking after a person with Dementia is not like nurturing a child who, every day, exhibits a greedy appetite for life. Everything about my mother speaks to decay, to dying. A banana in a fruit bowl blackening. Its rot observed by a time-lapse camera.

2008

I bought new shoes that day, that day back then.

They were ridiculously high. Six inches, at least.

I never wear heels. I don't have the need: I live in bare feet, the only thing between my soles and the floor a slippery talc of dust.

'Where on earth will you wear them?' my head demanded. 'What a waste,' it tutted.

But I bought heels that day anyway. My heart wasn't listening.

I laughed as I tried them on, teetering around a store. Some observers smiled, some looked on po-faced: I was too old to be lurching, giggling across a shop floor to the amusement of my then eleven-year-old daughter.

'Go on Mum! Get them!' urged Hat.

I was shorter by then than my two eldest children. And smaller and lighter than my son, seventeen at the time. Once I could pick him up. Now, he could me; he swept me clean off my feet, held me in an embrace so tight he winded me with his man-child strength. And Amelia, willowy slender, clasped me so that my head fitted into the curve described by her shoulder and neck. My face beneath her chin. My complexion, lined and pummelled by the march of time, the tread of worrying about, and laughing with, three children, looked parchment-old against the smooth alabaster of her fourteen-year-old one.

Once it was I who lifted them, swung them upwards in dizzying circles, round and round, higher and higher, and shrieked 'Weeeeeee,' and then again, their delighted laughter an encore: 'Again, Mama, again!'

I didn't just buy heels so that I could smile at their expressions when they noticed my newfound elevation. (Which they did – then rushed to lift the hem of my trousers to expose my secret).

I bought heels so that I could buy some time. Fill a space again. So that – for the briefest time – I might feel the shape of their heads against my shoulder.

'Mind the gap, Mum,' Hat warned as I boarded the train, tottering tall and perilous.

* * *

Most nights while Amelia was in hospital, persuaded I ought to go home to my own bed, I'd wake hours before dawn, toss and turn, then I'd give up on sleep altogether and slide from the sheets. I would pull on yesterday's shorts and a t-shirt, pick up the car keys and my phone and slip out into the sultry darkness to drive to the hospital. I drove too fast on empty roads lit by a sagging moon and would barrel onto the wards to the surprise of the nurses who only expected me at breakfast time.

Too little sleep unpicks a person (sleep, which knits up the ravelled sleave of care, Shakespeare said). I could feel my voice rising hysterically as I fretted to the doctors that the meds weren't doing what they needed to do fast enough. Or when my daughter's veins closed up, inflamed and blue, and nurses would have to prod for a new passage for the IV so bruises would bloom. I spent too much time hunched over my phone late at night, my haggard complexion jaundiced by the screen's glow, as I texted updates to family and friends.

I enraged Amelia's physician by asking, over and over, 'Are you sure this is the best antibiotic...?' until, one morning, worn down by my doubt and my questions, he shouted at me: 'Are you the medically qualified adult here, or am I?'

Which embarrassed my husband who lost patience with me: 'You are a great mother,' he said sternly, 'but sometimes you are Too Much.'

Too Much?

Too *much*!

My eyes welled hot tears behind sunglasses and I tilted my chin defiantly and didn't say a word.

It took me days to go back to this accusation, to unpack it: *sometimes you are Too Much.*

My mother would not have done what I did. She would not have questioned the doctors. She would not have doubted them. She would not have gone behind their backs, researching the medication her daughter had been prescribed. She would not have dreamt of speaking to other doctors in other hospitals because she was not confident the drug regime being administered to her daughter in that hospital was the right one.

She would not have slid out of the bed she shared with her husband, pulled on a pair of shorts and driven to the hospital in the middle of the night.

She would not have catastrophised. But nor would she have fought the system as I did; she'd have agreed with every opinion, consented politely to every decision made with regards her daughter's care. My mother would not have been the pain in the hospital's arse that I became.

I don't know if that means she would have been any better under the same circumstances.

Did I achieve faster results because of the way I am? Did Amelia recover more quickly because of that? Would her hospital experience have been calmer had I been? I don't know.

*

Donald Winnicott was an English paediatrician and psychoanalyst who understood the balancing acts of mothers.

He delivered over sixty broadcasts on *Woman's Hour.* His theme: a mother need only be good enough. He acknowledged parenting meant failing. He understood mothering was difficult and isolating and that it was enough to love your child most of the time, but that it was also normal to need to vent: 'Damn you, you little bugger,' he said.

A Good Enough mother was, he concluded, good enough. Imperfect parenting could be a positive thing, he believed.

Even in her illnesses, even in the emotional absences these have sliced – her distance with Depression, her disappearing with Dementia – Mum gifted us something of substance.

In Depression she shared her library of books – *Malignant Sadness, Noonday Demon, Sunbathing in the Rain* so that I could hold in my hand something that weighted this most slippery of maladies, so that I might understand a tiny part of the place she was at a loss to describe.

Later, in Dementia, she answered all my questions until she could not; Depression had seasoned my courage to ask them:

'Do you mind the forgetting, Mum?' I asked her.

'Not really,' she said, 'I just worry people will think I am stupid when I cannot remember.'

Imperfect parenting. A good enough mother: *'It's what mother octopuses do: they put everything into brooding their young and then they die.'*

★

A long time later – after all this – when I'm sharpening my memories on the whetstone of my mother's blunted ones, I will realise – again – that it was precisely where she lost her strength that her children found theirs. I will know that in her sometimes absences – because the black dog had sunk its teeth into her and dragged her off into a dark corner where we could not reach her, or because Dementia meant she forgot us – she left us something precious and lasting.

Years ago, for a piece I was writing for a newspaper, I had cause to interview a Californian man whose job it was to counsel the super-wealthy on how to bring their children up without spoiling them. He said parents needed to build children with backbone: to pander to every whim, shield them from all life's blows, would be to reduce them to the consistency of over-cooked spaghetti, 'Too soft. No spine, see,' he said.

'What should we be looking to raise our children as, then?' I asked.

'Violin strings,' he said, without a moment's hesitation, 'strong, resistant, able to spring back into shape.'

My siblings and I resonate with a song of resourcefulness. I know this now.

★

My children's father is the financial glue of this home: he has supported good educations. He has paid for doctors' appointments, the orthodontist, holidays. He budgets and plans and manages logistics with the necessary cold eye of reason and with the backup of a spreadsheet. He is the sensible counter to all my drama and distress and wild dreams.

He is the tangible ballast at the bottom of this ship, keeping it afloat. He is the protective hull, keeping us contained, a roof over our heads.

What, then, am I?

Am I its bow? Do I ease my children's passage through the world? An anchor at the end of the day, tethering them to all that is safe and known? Or could I be the ship's bridge, the point from which they can navigate a way through their worlds?

Or must I be the wind in their sails? Urging, endorsing, encouraging them on?

I am all of these.

And when my mother was plain sailing under blue skies, when she wasn't stalled by the doldrums, she was too.

2022

We are in the car; we are zipping along a ribbon of grey asphalt which I can see sweating in temperatures that soar above 30 degrees. The scrub roadside is a sage blur, hills on the horizon are smudged by white heat so that their profiles are blunt and ashen. This road is as familiar to me as a loved one's face: I grew up not far from here, I have driven it a hundred times. I know the sweep of it, which mountains to expect when, which once-small towns bloom where and which have exploded so that the surrounding plains are patchworked with the silver of corrugated iron roofs.

My phone lies in my palm. I turn it over every now and again and surreptitiously refresh the page I have open – a flight tracker site: I am watching my eldest daughter's descent into London. She is six minutes away from landing. I have followed her passage since last night, when she left us. Three flights later and she is almost there. I have checked the take-off and landing of every single one.

Ant, driving, begins to tell me a story. He once rode this road on his motorbike, he says. He was 22. He did the 450-mile trip wearing shorts, a pair of flip-flops, his head bare of crash helmet, a friend as passenger. They only stopped once in fourteen hours – for breakfast and a beer.

'Didn't you even wear a hat?' I ask.

'Not even a hat,' he laughs.

I smile. But secretly I am horrified, 'What did your mum think?'

He shrugs, 'I don't know.'

She mightn't even have known he was riding home to see her, he says.

She'd have been pleased to see him, I know that. But I also know – because I knew her – that there would have been no fuss on his arrival, no interrogation as to his journey or the reckless nature of it, no reprimands. She'd have greeted him with a kiss, 'Hello darling,' she'd have smiled, 'good trip?'

And he'd have limped in with his sore seat from sitting so

long, and his red face. He'd have slung an arm around her shoulder, 'Great trip, Mum, cup of tea?'

Sometimes I want to be her, I want to be *that* mother. I want not to be forever braced for some impact cast of my imagination. I want not to expect the worst. I want to allow my children the space to have adventures without breathing down their necks, sending messages demanding they update me on their progress, insisting they text me when they have arrived wherever it is they are going: from my sister's in Wiltshire back to London, home after a late night out, or that they've landed safely after flying across the world.

I sneak a sly peek at my phone again.

(Sometimes you are Too Much).

My daughter's flight landed nine minutes ago. Ahead of time.

She will text me shortly. She will say, 'Here safe and sound, Mum, just waiting for my bag, love you x'

She will do this because she knows me.

My son does not tell me some things for the same reason. Years later, travelling in southeast Asia, he takes a boat trip which he knows I am anxious about. He wrote in a message to my sister, 'I told Mum the trip was tomorrow so she would not worry today.'

When Hattie moves to South America for a year, I almost add a tracking app to her phone, so that I can see where she is, make sure she is always within my virtual sights. But at the last minute I resist the urge. And then, ironically, when Hattie is attacked on a Santiago street late at night, when she is punched in the face so that blood spills, when her phone, her passport, all her bank cards are stolen at the same time, I know nothing. I sleep on and only know of the incident when her older sister calls me the next day.

She prefaces the news with, 'Hat is fine, do not panic, but…'

What could I have done anyway?

'Why do you always imagine the worst?' my husband asks with the click of irritation.

Yes. Why? Is it because I know that life can suddenly grow turbulent, a mirror-flat sea unruffled by even the tiniest swell until it is made tempestuous by storm, its satin surface torn by the rip of currents and the weft of waves? Is it because my own life was sideswept when I least expected it?

I'm so sorry; he's dead.

2022 (After)

You wonder how, don't you, you wonder how an illness could shear your children from you. What sickness could bear such devastating pathology that it would sever your children? Slice right through the emotional umbilicus that binds you – has bound you tightly for so many years. It seems – seemed – unthinkable.

When Mum comes to live with me, a lot of her stuff comes too, including piles of correspondence between us. Piles. I am astonished at envelopes full of my letters to her, airmail paper that has grown silken and soft with age. We were written into each other's lives in every way – on the page and in our DNA. Where did that go?

How can a disease be the undoing of biology?

How can my mother not remember me?

'Do you know,' Mum says with a conspiratorial grin and a twinkle in her eye, 'she' (indicating my sister) 'has been telling me tall tales again?'

'Yes?'

'She says she is my *daughter*,' and Mum roars with laughter.

'Well, she's *my* sister.'

Mum stops laughing and looks at me. Her expression says: 'And? So?'

'Well. *I'm* your daughter. So if she's my *sister*, she must be your daughter too.'

Mum is aghast: 'No you're not,' she says.

And she presents an argument to explain why we absolutely cannot be her daughters:

'I would never have chosen *your* names for *my* children.'

There is a small sneer to her tone – *your* names.

When I relate this exchange to my best friend, Caroline, she says, I wonder what your mum would have said if you'd asked what names she'd have chosen.

And I will always wish afterwards that I had posed the question.

⋆

These conversations spin as farce, because Mum insists on winning the argument (another new facet to my mother's Dementia-distorted character: the determination to win an argument, the will to argue at all and I admit to feeling delighted by this): 'How come then, in all the years I've been visiting you, you've never told me, *not once*, that you are my daughter?'

Do you see this catastrophic leak of logic – the ship's going down – as if we must tell our mothers we are their daughters? This thing is much bigger than just the lost memory that I am.

Also: *Visiting you?*

She *lives* with me.

There are no answers. I give up.

My husband wants to know why I press this fact of kinship. His the easy position of one whose parents were never drowned out by Dementia.

'I want her to know she has children, children who care, who will look after her,' I say, for I imagine it would be terrifying to know you had children but did not know where those children were. (I am that mother who wanted to put a tracking app on her adult daughter's cell phone, remember?).

When I ask Mum where her children are, not only does she not know, but she doesn't seem to care.

She shrugs, 'Somewhere in Africa, I suppose?'

All she does know is that, today, I'm not one of them.

After

Sometimes, when my children were little, when days went wrong – were filled with frustration, tears, cross words – at the end of those days, as I watched their sleeping faces, small expressions relaxed into angelic repose, guilt gnawed at me: would today have been easier if I'd been more patient, less irritable? Done things differently?

Would today have been a better day if I were a better mother?

I do that now: Consider the day retrospectively after I've helped Mum to bed in this peculiar new role where I must tend regressions which renders her not childlike but dependent upon me in the way a child would be.

I smear toothpaste on her toothbrush and monitor as she brushes, 'And the back ones,' I say. I remind her to have a wee and listen to the sound of her peeing and the satisfied sigh when she has, 'Finished,' she says. I help her into her nightdress: 'Arms up, Ma.'…

Some mornings, Mum is up before six and wondering where the rest of the house is.

'I have been up for hours,' she complains when I pop my head around her door. She wears a childish expression then – the thrust of her jaw, the infantile, obvious pout – 'All on my *own*! Where *were* you?'

'Mum, it's not even six.'

'It's not that early,' she snaps.

The watch I recently bought her – with its big, bold digits – is fastened uselessly about her thinning wrist. My purchase a pitiful representation of hope; she can't tell the time anymore.

And there, there it is again: the sameness. I taught my children to tell the time.

'When the big hand is here,' and I pointed at the twelve, 'and the little here, 7, then, THEN it's time to get up.'

I cannot teach Mum about big hands and little hands and the polite time to wake the house up.

She has drunk three cups of tea from a flask in her room already. No kettles. She boils them dry and trips the lights.

I don't shake the irritation from my voice fast enough: 'Mum! I've only just woken up!'

'Don't be nasty to me,' she whimpers, that defiant chin tucked in now, eyes downcast.

I check myself then, apologise, suggest she gets dressed, coax her out of her nightdress.

Arms up, Ma.

'Let her do it herself,' my subconscious tuts. But I have to get to work and Mum needs dressing, teeth-brushing, breakfast. I chivvy while trying to pretend I have all the time in the world. It's like walking into the wind; needing to be somewhere and never getting there.

Two steps forward, one back.

I watch Mum battling with a button on her blouse. I slow my breathing, count to ten, 'Can I help with that?' I ease feet into shoes. Watch as she struggles with the zip on her fleece, my fingers itch to do it up for her.

This is the pace of days with Dementia. Slow hours falter and slide, time is lost between gaps.

I hold her hand on a mid-morning walk. When did I stop holding my children's hands on a walk?

Two hours later, two hours when I cram in as much work as I can, I find Mum shuffling and furious.

'Why did you abandon me? You just *left* me,' she shouts, her voice rising and shrill, 'You just left me with all these people.'

'All these people?'

'All *these* people,' and she flaps a hand in the direction of something I cannot see, 'Waiting for the doctor; you were meant to come and get me, but you didn't.'

I am frantically playing catchup – *waiting for the doctor?* – trying to bridge a widening chasm between what's real, what's not.

All what people? Where?

And then it dawns on me: *Doc Martin*. That's it. I left her watching *Doc Martin*.

I left her separated from the imagined by a screen, a story held safely behind glass. I turn my back and it empties a fictional physician's patients into the room where she sits.

2022

One day, one particularly bad day, full of holes and lost things and confusion, I tried to explain a misunderstanding to my mother (as if she might make sense of her world if I could just tip it the right way up). But she just grew more and more agitated: Her comprehension of the situation we were stumbling over was entirely skewed.

'Don't lie to me!' she shouted.

She glared at me. Hot eyes; heated tones. I expected her to cry. Once she would have cried. Once she would never have invited this sort of row, never spoken to anybody like this. Once she would have apologised.

'How could my memory be so bad that I can't remember something as important as that?' she demanded.

She delivered this as a sort of triumphant finale: a rhetorical question that asked, 'What have you got to say for yourself *now?*'

But I do have something to say: 'Because, Mum, your short-term memory is gone.' Gone.

And then I say it. This word I have avoided using until now.

Backed into a corner, I am forced to explain, to use the D word where I'd always avoided it before.

(For what is worse – and I still do not know: that my mother thinks I am deceiving her or for me to tell her the truth, the whole, horrid truth of this?)

I hesitate a few moments and then, with a deep breath, 'You have Dementia, Mum.'

I say it very gently, as if in my casual namedrop delivery I might soften the blow. As if a lack of amplification might whisper it away.

The air in the room seems to still with silence; my own breath is stopped in my chest, I imagine the clock by Mum's bedside stops its ticking.

She looks shocked: 'Dementia? Dementia! That means I am demented, DEMENTED,' she cries.

And for a second I think of tribal communities in Namibia, in south-west Africa, where Dementia sufferers are labelled witches: Dementia from the Latin *demens*, 'out of one's mind.'

'No, no,' I protest. 'Not demented. Just a bit forgetful.'

'Just a bit forgetful': a euphemism to blunt the sharp edge of all this.

I never use the D word again. And soon, mercifully, she forgets I ever did.

★

Later, I help her shower, closing the curtain to preserve a shred of her dignity, to pretend it matters, I help her into a fresh nightgown, *arms up,* I tuck her in as I used to my children:

And then, 'Good night Mum, sleep tight, don't let the bugs bite.'

'Goodnight,' she smiles and, as an afterthought, 'What's your name again?'

'Anthea, it's Anthea.'

I close the door and lean against it, guilt swallows me.

Could I have been kinder? More patient? What could I have done differently?

Would today have been a better day if I were a better daughter?

★ ★ ★

There is a recognised phenomenon during pregnancy – micro-chimerism. I look up the etymological roots of *chimera* now. In Greek mythology, the chimera was a fire breathing female monster with a lion's head, a goat's body, a serpent's tail.

Micro-chimerism describes the two-way flow of cells between mother and foetus, when cells from the baby migrate towards the cells of the mother and settle into the many tissues of her body, including her brain. These cells accumulate during every pregnancy, and have been detected in a mother's blood many years later, as if the small signature of what – or who – was there is written indelibly within. As if for those women – those fierce, brave, fire-breathing women – who conceived babies but lost them, were never able to mother them, as if for them, their babies left an everlasting bruise.

Chimera, also: 'a thing which is hoped for but is illusory or impossible to achieve.'

I knew that mothers and their babies are connected in a million ways: from the umbilical cord that tethered them to one another and then wound its way outside the womb until they were separated for the first time. I knew they were intricately tied to one another by the helix ribbons of DNA, by all the tender familial links of a parent's siblings and their own, by emotion and memories and by story.

But I did not know, until now, that babies are connected most profoundly – the born, the unborn, those who predeceased their mothers – at a deep, sustaining cellular level: they were as one with their mothers.

And they always will be.

Even when their mothers forget them.

2021 (After)

'My son Rob says I have a daughter called Anthea. But I don't.'

Her voice trails off and in the delivery of her words, I hear her unspoken question: *Do I?*

'You do, Mum: that's me. I'm Anthea.' And then, to make myself feel better, to take the sting out of all this, so that we all feel better about Mum forgetting, I add, 'I'm your favourite child.'

I say it often. Sometimes Mum laughs.

Sometimes, if there's somebody else present who might be one of Mum's other children (who knows?) she says, 'Shhh, don't say it out loud or he/she' (gesturing the other party) 'might be hurt.'

And then the other party – my sister, my brother – fall about laughing and some part of Mum gets the joke and she laughs too.

Sometimes her old diplomatic self asserts itself: 'I don't have favourites; I love you all the same.'

Today she just says, 'Oh,' in a small voice. And I don't know if the 'oh' is because she understands she has forgotten something significant.

Or because she has a daughter called Anthea.

I tell my sister in a voice note. Why does it feel like a confession – this owning up to Mum not remembering me though she knew – that day – my brother? As if admitting to something I am ashamed of. Have I failed her in some way that she is erasing me first?

Then I do what I have done before. I tell my children:

Remember this. If I ever, ever forget you, know I have loved my children more than anything in the world.

My youngest messages back:

And so has Gran.

★

How do you remain tethered to a parent who is being erased by Dementia?

For that is what it feels like from where I stand – as if my mother is growing so insubstantial there is nothing to hold onto anymore.

And how do we – we who are well – hold that person's attention as their focus shifts, narrows, grows slippery with a landscape that is constantly changing?

'Where am I? Am I on a Ship? Who are you?'

Why a Ship? Is it the distancing disorientation of the disease that does this? Does she feel the ocean swell beneath her in increasingly precarious balance, as if trying to get her sea legs? When she tips, does she lose sight of the tenuous lie of land that she briefly held? Is that why she's always looking, always lost – *Where am I? Who are you?*

Is she getting smaller and smaller because she's receding from my view in all these changes that manifest: this is not the mother I knew. I am not the daughter she remembers.

Soon she'll float clean off the edge of my horizons.

Sometimes I reach out a hand to her, to check she is still here. She will register the gesture and reciprocate by patting my arm: 'All right, pet,' she'll say.

I notice a trend later as I flick through photograph albums.

In most of the pictures of Mum and me, I have draped an arm about her shoulders.

Or I have pinned both of her arms to her sides as I envelop her in both of mine, an embrace as I bring her in close.

Or I rest a hand upon her leg.

Or her arm.

Or I am holding her hand.

These were unconscious gestures. I wasn't aware of them at the time. But now, in this series of snapshots, pages of them, taken at a great distance in time over the years; I can find almost no photograph where Mum and I are not connected physically in the frame.

Was I instinctively reaching out to check she was there?

Was I holding on to her?

Was I reassuring, by touch: I am here?

Is this what I am doing now?

* * *

Slowly, the heat in Amelia's foot dissipates, her colour returns to normal, her complexion no longer bears the sheen of fever. And we are home. She is a long way off being well. She is weak and sore and can't walk. Her toe is hard and blackening and swollen. The doctors have warned recovery could take weeks. But I can breathe again.

Slowly I feel it is safe to tell a story, this story. With this ending. I can dip into the ether to take a peek at how much worse this could have been: she could have been stung on a more vulnerable part of her body – higher up could have implicated more organs, created respiratory problems, cardiac arrest even.

She could have been alone in that rising tide.

For two weeks after she is discharged from hospital, I share a bed with her so that I can count out my daughter's medication in the middle of the night, so that I can help her to the bathroom, so that I can have her close, so that I reach out in the dark and place my palm on her brow and reassure myself that she is cool and that the infection is being held at bay.

So that I can reassure her I am there. So that I can reassure myself she is here.

★

When Amelia is well enough to return to work, almost three weeks after she should have done, when she can bear a sock on her foot, can walk with crutches, dragging the affected foot and withered leg about behind her, I book her travel.

I lecture her on which meds to take when, during her thirteen-hour flight to London. I urge her to keep her foot up. I make her promise to see her GP and to keep an eye on her toe.

I am still doing these things when I hear the rumble of her taxi down the sandy road to the house, I see its headlights cast a glow against the windows. And a familiar weight settles in my chest.

'Time to go,' I say.

Cheerfully she parcels up chargers and phone and Kindle and stray bits of clothing to bung into a bursting suitcase. She hugs me. She tells me she loves me. I close the door of her taxi. I stand in my pyjamas and bare feet in the dark and I wave.

And it is then that I know I am not Too Much. For when I have to, when I know they are safe, well, happy – my children – I drop my arms from around them, I peel my clenched fists open, I kiss my fingertips and I blow.

I let them go.

Chapter 5: Learning to Swim

Learning to swim is a life-or-death skill, essential for every child.
United States Swim School Association

1971

My mother taught me to swim. She taught me in a borrowed pool whose sides were bearded with algae so that to touch the tiles was to stroke something silken – like wet down. The water in the pool was the colour of the sea, a soft, slow going-green. There were frogs which made me shudder and a ladder to climb down to a surface that was lower than it should have been; a hot sun and lazy maintenance had conspired to drink greedily. The ladder trembled as I climbed down, seized by fear and strummed by a thrill.

Mum said later that she taught me because she never swam with strength or confidence. She only swam because she felt duty-bound to encourage her children into the water and then to accompany them there when they – we – were little. When she swam, she held her head at an awkward angle, straining her neck so her face was as high above the waterline as possible, wincing and turning away from our splashing, 'Stop it,' she'd scold, 'Stop it.'

She was so afraid of putting her head under water she wouldn't wash her hair in the shower. She shampooed it at the sink. Later, her spine bent by osteoporosis and age, her shoulders rounded as a shell, hair washing is a challenge; it's hard to get her close enough to the basin so I can tip mugs of warm water over her head. She holds a flannel to her eyes, just as she encouraged us to do when she washed our hair as children. And just as she did then, I check every few minutes: 'You okay under there?' And I do something else she did then, too: I fashion her wet, sudsy hair into horns. 'You're a buffalo, Mum,' I laugh, and she does too. 'Or how about a unicorn?' I suggest as I scrape it together and mould it near her forehead. When we're done, I towel her head dry and apologise for her drenched collar, her sodden lap where suds have spilled.

She smiles, 'That doesn't matter,' she says.

But that day, that day when I was five, my mother stole courage from somewhere and, in haughty Lady Wilson's pool, she gave me my first swimming lesson. Lady Wilson, who was not in evidence that morning, acquiesced to our use of her pool because she could not resist my mother's charm and elegance which lent rare town-mouse chic to our ordinary farming community.

We were both a little shaky; I teetered on the lowest rung trying to pluck up courage as Mum tried to keep her balance on the bottom of the pool, which in a clean hotel pool would have winked sturdy encouragement but in this one I couldn't see, and my mother kept sliding on.

'Come on love,' she said, hands held out, smile broad, 'You can do it.'

I took a deep breath, braced myself for the cold and lunged from that wobbly ladder and into her arms – a leap of faith: I knew my mother would keep me afloat.

And my mother, my mother who hated the water, who never put her face beneath its surface, caught me in a firm, sure grip. Then she placed a palm under my tummy and urged me to paddle with my arms, 'like the dogs do,' and to kick with my legs: 'Harder, harder, good girl.'

And I – I who plough out fast and too far with strong, certain strokes now, I who dive so deep I can hear the sea's song above me – I learned to love it.

* * *

The irony of my mother's Depression is that it cultivated its counter in me. Where her illness blunted her profile, it sharpened mine; where it stalled her with lack of direction, it drove me; where it hollowed her with a redundancy, it filled me with occupation. And where it left her inert, it fuelled my energy. How it came about was entirely accidental but there must have been some latent understanding, some prickle beneath my skin that pinched me awake: *I must try do something so that what happened to Mum might not happen to me.*

2002

I remember when the project began to take shape. I remember that clearly. I remember that I turned to this task to fill days suddenly emptied of children as my youngest joined her siblings at school. The house was the quietest it had been in years.

I walked into my children's recently emptied bedrooms one morning and saw pyjamas tossed to the floor, evidence of hasty risings. I picked them up and tucked them under pillows. I hesitated before straightening a tangle of sheets. I laid my hand upon them and was sure they still held the warmth of young skin in their threads. I turned off lights left burning and closed doors and still the silence shouted back.

I sat at the kitchen counter consumed by disorientation. Loss of direction. Loss of definition.

Just loss, really Mum had said.

I began to cry. My husband looked on nervously.

'What's the matter?' he asked.

'I don't know what to do next.'

My husband is a practical man.

He thought for a moment and then he said: 'Make jam?'

Make jam? *Make jam!*

I was indignant that he presumed knocking up preserves would be enough to fill days empty of the demanding insistence of small children.

So I didn't make jam. I mean I did. I do, badly so that either it won't set at all and slips and slides all over your plate and cannot be spread obediently on toast. Or else I overcook it so it cements itself inside the jar and won't be coaxed out.

Instead I began to write, a messy, sort of metaphorical jam making.

★

Why words, though?

Perhaps it began in the library of books Mum collected, books that described the rawness of madness through the experiences of those whose lives had been abraded by it, books which lent a lens so that she might see how others had lived with it. Perhaps Mum hoped that within these stories she would find the answers that eluded her. Perhaps somebody else's Beginning would lend insight into her own. Perhaps somebody else's Middle would reassure her she was not alone. I know she hoped in their Endings there would be answers.

Maybe just the fact of reading about a life that matched her own, where she could identify some part of her lost self, made her feel less isolated, because here was the proof: There were others who understood the weight of this incorporeal thing.

Maybe that's why I began to read the same books? To witness their weight – to hold in my hand hundreds of pages bound sturdily by a hard cover was to conjure something of substance of this invisible sickness. If it was written down – there, see? – in black and white, it *must* be real.

Resorting to the written word in search of answers or succour was instinctive: 'Read a book,' Mum said when we were little and complained of being bored. Read a book when there was nothing else to do and when there was so much else to be done that you needed an excuse to escape. 'Read a book to find out,' Mum instructed, so that the arrival of fifteen volumes of *The New Universal Library,* with their turquoise covers and embossed gold lettering, felt like having the world at my fingertips, the answer to any question I might ask.

I look up 'Depression' now in Vol 4, *Col – Dri*, and Page 343 delivers a choice: which 'Depression' do you want to know about? Depression as economics, Depression as meteorology or Depression as psychology? Depression as a homonym, I think, which strikes me as apt, given the way the illness sliced my mother into different parts of her thinning self. And then sliced her again.

The edition, open on my desk now, the same desk where I began to pot words more than twenty years ago, is open for the first time in decades ('We have Google now,' my children tell me when I suggest they conduct their own research in the same pages.)

The scent of old paper fills my nostrils, the page feels floury, the language dates back to the year I was born. As my children observe – this is how we looked things up in the Olden Days.

Involutional melancholia, I read, *occurs with the onset of the menopause, when the decline in the female sex organs frequently causes a loss of purpose in life.*

I snap the book shut crossly.

But then I remember: that's why I began to write, beginning with describing what it felt like on the outside as I grew to understand something of the experiences of those on the inside: I was afraid of losing my *purpose in life.*

So I read and re-read the stories of William Styron, who helped to illuminate the gloom with his *Darkness Visible*; Lewis Wolpert, who described how this horrible illness mutated in his *Malignant Sadness*; and Andrew Solomon, who laid the bones of it bare in his *Anatomy of Melancholy.*

These writers were able to articulate what my mother didn't always have the words to express.

But I still have questions. I will write and ask them myself, I think.

⋆

The first person I write to is Lewis Wolpert. Wolpert, who said Depression is 'sadness gone wrong,' described his experience of the illness as the worst of his life, 'More terrible even than watching my wife die of cancer'.

He urges me to keep writing, to express my own understanding of Depression.

I write to Gwyneth Lewis who wrote *Sunbathing in the Rain.* She tells me she knows exactly what I mean about my mother being able to cope with big things but not little ones, 'I am the same,' she says.

I tug titles off Mum's shelves and I track down the authors and I write, and I write, and I write.

I ask myself just once: am I really only doing this to give new purpose to my life? Or am I doing it because to see my mother's Depression articulated by academics and poets lends it palatable creativity? I tell myself it does not matter.

Carolyn Slaughter, writer turned psychotherapist, shares experiences with me: she grew up with a mother who battled with Depression; she grew up in Africa, a childhood she describes in her memoir, *Before the Knife*. She learned to make sense of her relationship with madness through language, she tells me. Her words endorse my efforts to do the same though I can't decide whether I hope that in pinning Depression's characteristics to a page, I will imprison it there where I can keep a close eye on it. Or because in articulating my understanding of the illness, I will understand my mother – and myself – better. Slaughter tells me 'if you can stand to sit with your mother's Depression and know it's not yours, and make a clear decision not to follow her into the dark, I guarantee it will not happen to you. But the acceptance of who she is and what she has is crucial to this process.'

And so I sit as close to Depression as I dare. I sit so close I can feel the cold rise from it. And I start to write down the answers to my questions.

For there will always be answers in words: Mum taught me that.

⋆ ⋆ ⋆

I do not remember a time when I didn't swim afterwards.

And every body of water I swam in describes a different part of my life, so that I sought them out – those pools, that sea – in order that I might dive in and swim my way to stilled thoughts. Or plough up and down arms thrashing, legs kicking, heart pumping, breaths measured so that, at the end of a burst of lengths, I pant hard and feel high on the rush.

I swam my way through a difficult relationship with food so that my flat tummy caved in and my costume was strung like a hammock between my hips. Sometimes I swam through hunger. I swam through the strange newness of boarding school in England. I swam through my first confusing winter there when the familiarity of the community pool, with its humid embrace and eye-stinging chlorine, seemed like companionship. The underwater sounds of that pool were the same as they were in pools everywhere, I could have been anywhere: the thrash of limbs, the muted voices on the water's edge, the distant hum of the paraphernalia that keeps pools clean. Except Lady Wilson's, of course.

I swam in London. My first job. My best friend, Caroline, and I found a pool in Mayfair of all places, the rarefied centre of an alien city. A lucky discovery. The price of a swim just a pound. The elderly, liveried doorman would smile at us, doff his cap and then lean hard into the heavy brass and wood portal that opened from a quiet street off a leafy square to let us in.

The pool was galleried beneath a vaulted ceiling, graceful poolside pillars were necklaced with greenery, the lighting muted. There were no children shrieking in this pool. There was almost nobody in it but us – sometimes just me. Me and the fencers, dancing muted steps away from one another's foils in some ancient choreography: *En garde! Prêts? Allez!*

I swam through my pregnancies. Settling my swollen body into water carefully, lowering myself until my belly and my baby were submerged. I felt lighter then. People remarked on arms tanned and taut, muscles that popped when I lifted anything: of course, I was pulling the weight of two of us through the water. I dove deep and propelled myself on a single breath from one end of the pool to the other, watching the last inhalation I took before I went under escape from me, a necklace of glass beads strung all the way to the surface. And then I would roll onto my back, my glorious mound a floating island and I would watch the excited wriggling of my unborn, undulations beneath my skin – a heel here, an elbow there.

All my children love to swim. They learned in the womb, kicking and twisting in an amniotic aquarium, little human fish anchored safely to their mother.

Later I swam my way through the faraway years of an outpost life; when all my children had left home for school or university and I found myself high and dry. I swam then. Hard. Fast. Every day. Twice a day. When isolation threatened to overwhelm, I drowned it out. I slipped into the pool at first light, my skin, chilled by dawn air, was blanketed beneath blood-warm water. An embrace; it felt like climbing into myself. I watched the sun caress the eastern edge of the sky until it blushed with pleasure as I stroked my way up and down and up and down.

My mother, who hated to put her head under water, who will not even stick it beneath the shower to wash her hair, taught me that was where I could go to gather myself. Underwater, where I can collect my thoughts, where my words line up, where I can swim out frustration or disappointment or fury.

And underwater I make a surprising discovery; you cannot cry if you're sitting at the bottom of a pool. The weight of water upon you won't let you leak tears. And weeping requires the fuel of oxygen. The physics thwarts the physical.

But you can scream.

I sank to the bottom and opened my mouth and let out a roar and the water muffled my anguish. In water I feel peeled back. As if my fluid self meets liquid and I am made stronger in that union. And I am more graceful in water than I am on dry land. On land I run with ungainly stride, I dance without rhythm. But underwater? Underwater I am lithe and swift and graceful.

And I always emerge feeling braver.

How strange that being underwater helps me feel grounded.

2021 (After)

Mum and I are sitting in my sister's small sunlit summer garden when Mum says something unexpected, out of the blue, so that I will puzzle afterwards: what prompts these sudden thoughts; memories which rise as flotsam, small unbroken parts from the wreckage of her intellect?

'I don't know why my parents never sent me to university. I was clever enough; I should have gone. My life might have been quite different.'

My mother has never expressed this regret. Ever.

'I'm sorry, Mum,' I say, 'What would you have liked to have studied, if you had gone to university?'

'I don't know. Perhaps I'd have become a teacher.'

'You would have made an excellent teacher, Mum – you taught us kids.'

Us Kids. As if she might remember.

She smiles but looks blank; no, she does not remember. She does not remember the parcels of books that arrived by train.

She does not remember delivering Correspondence School lessons on joined-up writing as she placed her hand over our small ones to guide pencils gripped tight (so that small calluses would swell on the middle finger of my right hand) as we tracked a row of cursive c's on baking parchment for tracing paper. She does not remember teaching my brother and me to read as we swung bare feet above hot dogs panting, sprawled starfish to cool on cement floors. She does not remember our childish astonishment at the implausibility of Janet and John's socks-and-shoes world where rivers ran gin-clear and a dog called Pat never needed picking of ticks.

She does not remember.

'And then you helped me teach my own kids,' I nudge.

No. Still nothing. No sweet recollections of introducing my son to arithmetic, not in a textbook, but through the medium of play: an ingenious game she invented using bottle tops as coins and urging her grandson to buy the items she'd arranged in her 'shop'. She does not share my precious memory of him counting out Coca-Cola tops to buy back a book he already owned, his careful concentration, his delight when he got it right and Mum swept him into a congratulatory hug.

She does not remember that maths remains my son's strongest subject.

But what she does remember is that her father was a doctor.

'I could even have become a doctor. Like Dad,' Mum continues now, 'I think it would have been good if I'd done something else, perhaps it would have helped, at times, when things were difficult, you know,' and she falters, her voice trails off as a brief shadow bruises her face, as if trying to recall some unhappy fudgy memory, 'I had nothing to do when my children grew up, you see.'

She speaks to me as if I'm not one of them.

This is why, this is where, Depression slunk in. It found a gap, somewhere to get a toehold, to put down those long parasitic roots that spread later as devil's guts; strangle-weed; witch's hair. If Mum had kept busy, would her brain have been able to keep busy later? Can we bank knowledge like we can a library of encyclopaedias so it's always to hand? Are occupation and engagement the fuel and lubricating oil that keep engines of cognition running smoothly, even in age?

'Use it or lose it,' the experts warn: don't let those engines idle.

⋆

Dr David Merrill, an adult and geriatric psychiatrist and director of the Pacific Brain Health Center tells me, 'If you're looking to build physiological muscle, you might up the ante; if you're a regular walker, say, you may start to walk further, faster, more frequently.' The same applies to our brains, he says, they respond to workouts, too, just like any other part of our body. 'The "use it or lose it approach" is not just a hypothesis, it's a basic biologic fact that holds as true for our brains as for our muscles or our bones.'

'You could have been an Olympic athlete,' he says, 'but if you don't keep up your physical fitness, you'll get out of shape. The same is true for synapse counts and cell numbers in the aging brain – ongoing environmental enrichment matters. Even if you're college-educated and worked in an intellectually challenging environment during early to middle adulthood, if you don't keep up the cognitive stimulation as you get older, there will be significant decline.'

Brain imaging illustrates this point: learning and engagement contribute towards preservation of brain volumes and help prevent, or slow, the shrinking of memory centres in much the same way as physical exercise keeps our visible muscle in well-defined shape. Experts refer to this phenomenon as 'cognitive reserve', defined as 'A property of the brain that allows for better-than-expected function given the degree of adverse brain related change.'

Merrill says the phrase makes him think of a financial savings account for retirement.

It makes me think of something life-sustaining saved for later, a dam against the emptying drought of Dementia: a reservoir.

The phrase, 'cognitive reserve,' was coined by Professor Yaakov Stern, a neuropsychologist and chief of the Cognitive Neuroscience Division in the Department of Neurology at Columbia University.

Stern published a paper in the early Nineties that observed people with higher education were less likely to develop the symptoms of Alzheimer's Disease. When he presented it at the Academy of Neurology, friends and colleagues made fun of the idea. 'It seemed so far-fetched,' he remembers, 'that something like education could counter the plaques and tangles of Alzheimer's.'

Stern used 'cognitive reserve' to differentiate it from the 'brain reserve' described by Robert Katzman a few years previously. Katzman published research in the late-Eighties based on the examination of the brains of a number of elderly residents in a care home. He found some of these people's brains showed significant pathology of Alzheimer's yet their cognition ranked in the top 20 per cent of the nursing home residents, as good as, or better, than residents without any brain pathology.

Katzman concluded that this was because these people had bigger, heavier brains bearing a higher number of neurons and synapses; they had more brain to start with, ergo had more 'brain reserve' to lose in the face of Dementia.

Katzman was a pioneer in the field of Alzheimer's; his work demonstrated how widespread the condition was. When he published research on the prevalence of the illness in China, he concluded that people with higher levels of education appeared to have lower incidence of Dementia.

When he read this, Stern assumed the findings were flawed, 'I thought it must be a mistake; they were using a mental status exam and I felt sure – of course – that people with higher education would do better on that test, I felt it needed an incidence study – starting with people who were not demented and following them over time.'

And so Stern and his team set out to do exactly that and found that people with less than eight years of education had twice the risk of developing Dementia as compared to those with more. They also found that people with 'low lifetime occupational attainment' bore a similar risk. The implication of these findings, Stern concluded, was that 'educational and occupational experiences imparted a reserve against the expression of Alzheimer's pathology.'

Why, though? How could education, topping up that cognitive reserve, protect you from the devastating symptoms of Dementia even in the face of pathology?

Each circuit in the brain develops as you learn new things, and as you learn new things, you are reinforcing existing connections as if flexing a muscle and making it stronger. Neurons involved in that learning create – and keep creating – *dendritic* (from the Greek *dendron*, tree) spines to communicate with other neurons. The more spines, the better the connectivity so when you are faced with degenerative brain processes, it takes longer to disconnect.

I think of the battery terminals in a car. If a vehicle has sat too long doing nothing, going nowhere, corrosion builds up which weakens the connection between terminal and cable: the message to start can't get through.

The brain's ability to reinforce connections – to *grow* connections – is described as neuroplasticity, and derives from the brain's innate and efficient ability to reorganise itself in order to accomplish tasks in the most efficient way using the least number of processes necessary.

'Highways,' one young scientist told me, 'are a great analogy to use in demonstrating cognitive reserve: if you only know one way home, and if for any reason that road is disrupted, that's it. No getting home. However, if through experience, *learning*, you have identified *five* routes home, and they're all active and you use all five, you are constantly reinforcing those routes so if one highway is damaged, by injury, illness, ageing, you can still get the message across, still communicate from one area of the brain to another. Still get home.'

Cognitive reserve is based on the understanding that the brain learns to use alternative neural networks in still-healthy regions.

We used to think that neuroplasticity was a privilege of youth, the same scientist says, 'But evidence over the last few years shows there is neurogenesis during adulthood and old age, just not at the same rate.' This was illustrated in research by neuroscientist Professor Eleanor Maguire at University College London. Her study of black-cab drivers in London showed that the area of the brain dedicated to location grew substantially when drivers learned 'The Knowledge'. This is ranked amongst the most difficult tests in the world and requires drivers to remember the names of 25,000 streets and landmarks across the capital.

But it isn't just formal education that banks cognitive reserve. Novelty does. As we get older, we tend to do the same things the same way over and over. So go somewhere new by a different route, one doctor urged.

Reading builds reserve as well because it requires you to understand all the words, follow the story, hold the plot in your head. Playing a musical instrument can, too, speaking more than one language does; bilingualism strengthens connections between different parts of the brain as you switch between languages. In old age, the frontal lobes begin to fail. If these have a good working relationship with other parts of the brain, a person can work around deficiencies to compensate for them.

Even something as simple as keeping a diary could have far-reaching effects.

Merrill tells me about the Nun Study, a ground-breaking analysis of 678 Catholic sisters between the ages of 75 and 107 who offered their brains for autopsy post-mortem.

On analysis, a number of the nuns' brains were full of the amyloid plaques characteristic of Alzheimer's disease. But it was not this fact which predicted whether they had suffered symptomatically in life with the memory loss and general befuddlement that characterises my mother now. What predicted that was their attitude to life and the complexity of their writing and journaling. In other words, said Merrill, the level of cognitive reserve they had built up to combat the accumulation of Dementia pathology later.

Epidemiologist David Snowdon, who conducted the study, described one of the nuns, Sister Mary, 'A remarkable woman who had high cognitive test scores before her death at 101 years of age. What is more remarkable is that she maintained this high status despite having abundant neurofibrillary tangles and senile plaques, the classic lesions of Alzheimer's disease.'

I look at Mum and know her cognitive reserve was drained by many things. Depression opened the floodgates. In my mind's eye I see the last of something precious rushing towards a giant plughole, the whirl of what is left spins in ever decreasing circles, faster and faster, the last bits of her caught like leaves as water vanishes down a drain.

Leaves for feathers.

And it's gone.

2009

One day I noticed the aquamarine from a ring my grandmother had given me was missing: the stone had gone and in its place, a naked silver mount. My grandmother was gifted the ring, with its sea-stone, in India. Sailors wore aquamarines for protection and to inspire courage.

When she gifted it to me as her eldest grandchild, I felt like the guardian of history, sentinel of something long past and precious. I panicked when I found the stone gone. I stripped. I climbed into the pool for the third time that day. I sank down to the bottom as if dropped by a trawler and I dredged, up and down, and there it was, blue on blue. A glassy eye blinking in the sun. I swept it up and climbed out and swaddled the stone in cotton wool. As soon as I could, I took the ring to a jeweller and instructed that he please recast the ring so that it was captured for good.

I twist it on my finger now. Sometimes I drop it into an inch of gin to clean it. When I put it back on, it gleams and I smell a little like I've had too much to drink. 'Mother's ruin,' Gran would have said, dragging on a cheroot.

She loved to swim too. If my mother took me swimming that first time, my grandmother kept taking me. And she kept swimming until she was in her eighties, when her body was hobbled by all kinds of decrepitude but her mind still tack-sharp. She would lower herself into the pool and leave her broken self on the edge, she would thrust herself out into the water and swim length after length in her inimitable, elegant side stroke. She only stopped swimming when somebody at the local pool tried to shove their way past her towards the showers and made a comment about old ladies being too slow. Slow, certainly, her sight going, Gran could still hear a pin drop. And she heard that.

She came home and cried. Imprisoned by fading vision and lameness, it was her swimming that set her briefly free. I tried hard to persuade her back to the pool.

But she never went again.

2023 (After)

I am walking with Mum. She wants to know what I have been doing all day.

'Working,' I say.

'Working! What do you do?'

'I'm a journalist,' I tell her.

She has no memory of all the stories I have written, no recollection of the day we sat in a garden and posed for a photographer from *The Times* because the paper was running the third story I had submitted on Depression.

I wrote hundreds of words on it, dozens of pieces and every retelling revealed something new about the shape of this thing; a scientist holding a specimen's skull aloft and inspecting it from every angle and in every light.

It was Mum who urged me to write about it then: 'If you don't write about it, how will people understand it?'

'Is that hard,' she asks, 'being a journalist?'

'Sometimes,' I say, 'When I can't find a good angle or the right words, then it can be frustrating.'

'But you don't give up?'

'No, Mum. I don't give up; I can't.'

Sometimes I drive my family mad with my inability to give up – on an appliance I can't fix, on a problem that needs solving, on an ailment that needs a cure: 'Just leave it' my husband begs. But giving up comes with risk. I know this.

Mum sighs: 'I think that's where I went wrong,' she says, 'I think I always gave up too soon.'

Where do these thoughts come from? These thoughts that swim to the surface so that – for a moment – she can skim them from the soup that's left of her brain? And how come she's never articulated them before? Is it because they weren't there? Or is it because they couldn't get through until Dementia gouged big holes in a filter made too fine by old fashioned manners, gender, a 1950s upbringing?

1986 (Before)

My mother applied to the Open University in the months after my father died and embarked on an Arts foundation course.

She unpacked her books when they arrived in the post, tidying titles away into shelves, labelling folders. I'd done the same at school, revelled in the newness of empty exercise books and pens still full of ink whose ends had not been chewed yet. I would inhale the scent of an open book, its pages not yet marked by fingers or notes or folded dog-eared at their corners. I would press them flat on my desk so that I heard their spines crack.

I watched Mum do the same now.

But not for long; she found home-learning isolating. Once the books were shelved there was anti-climax, and it was always in that oxygen-stealing anti-climax that the seeds of the next Depression took root and began to grow and suffocate enthusiasm.

I don't think she opened any of her books on the Renaissance, their backs remained unbroken and the pages unblemished by a single pencil stroke.

'Perhaps I need people?' she posed. But, by then, it was too late – for anything.

When she was better, she considered night classes.

'Perhaps if I'm learning *with* people?' she wondered, hopefully.

'What will you learn, Mum?' I asked her.

She looked up at me from where she sat at the dining table leafing through a pile of adult education prospectuses. The wood of the table gleamed with a recent polish so that it mirrored Mum's good spirits. Morning sunshine streamed through the windows, and herded dust motes into bright clouds.

And she smiled, 'I'm not sure,' she said, 'Maybe another language.'

'Or,' she pondered, turning a page to peruse the other courses on offer, 'I could do car maintenance?'

It's my turn to smile now, at the thought of her covered in engine oil and dressed in overalls as Dad used to be on the farm. We both knew it wasn't keeping a car going that was important, it was keeping her going that was.

In the end, though, Mum didn't sign up for anything. She went temping in the local industrial park instead and I tried not to mind when she told me she'd spent a whole day addressing envelopes.

When she got sick again she miserably observed, 'I wish I'd signed up for assertiveness classes.'

2017

When I was 51, I was accepted onto an MA in Creative Non-Fiction Writing at the Open University. I fought my way onto it. To register I was obliged to hold an undergraduate degree which I do not have. My application took the form of an essay:

> *So, the gatekeepers who stand at the river I am trying to forge, who guard the stepping stones, put a hand up when I stretch ahead of myself (such impertinence!) and try to clamber on to the rock marked MA Creative Writing.*
>
> *'You can't go there,' they say. 'You need to spend time on rock BA first.'*
>
> *'I don't want to,' I say.*
>
> *'Those are the rules,' they insist.*
>
> *'But I want to be on the MA,' I say.*
>
> ***It is expected that your spoken and written English will be of an adequate standard for postgraduate study. Please see the website for details.***
>
> *But it is, I say. And I have: looked at the website. I have written at* The Times, *the* Telegraph, *the* Washington Post. *In English. I know how to write, how to spell. I even know when to use 'affect' and when to use 'effect'.*
>
> *Nobody's listening.*
>
> ***If you do not have a background in creative writing, you are strongly recommended to undertake some preparatory work.***

I have! I have written at The Times, *the* Telegraph, *the* Washington Post. *In English...*

The MA in creative writing assumes that a candidate for a master's degree already has the knowledge and skills usually acquired by pursuing the subject at undergraduate level.

Why? Why does an undergraduate degree prove I have an aptitude for this course? Why does the experience I have gained, the lessons I've learned, the commitment I've shown, the work I've already done not count?

This is a module for candidates with experience of writing creatively and not for those who are just starting to write.

Oh please! Please listen to me: I write. I do. I promise! I have been writing for years, nearly twenty years. I understand the challenge of finding the right word, of testing it out, like a piece in a jigsaw puzzle: will it fit? I know the frustration of tossing it aside when it doesn't, feel the fat satisfaction when it does. I see language in colours and shapes, there are words, single words, that I love for their vibrancy, their flamboyance, their sheer brilliance, their fizz, the glorious way they roll from my tongue: words like 'onomatopoeia'. I know the thrill that comes with reading a phrase that has used language so economically, that every single word bears significance so that a short, unassuming sentence is lent telling weight.

The qualification will not offer remedial training for those who have an inappropriate undergraduate degree or inadequate experience.

I know that. It's also why I know this course is exactly right for me: no other course lends the opportunity to explore my passion in these genres: creative non-fiction and poetry. No other course affords the indulgence of a sometimes-compromised imagination but allows a delight in lyricism.

Any such students beginning the qualification do so at their own risk.

Is this a risk? If it is, it's a tiny one. Writing to that very first editor, with my ill-formed pitch, with no knowledge of how to interview a subject, no idea of how to navigate a style guide and only knowing I couldn't ask any of those questions. Now that was a risk.

So, I ask: have I proved myself adequate as a writer? Have I demonstrated competence? Do I have experience? Does that mean I bear the necessary qualification, the crutch to navigate my way from where I stand to the stone I've got my sights on, pushing my way past the first?

I am granted access to the course.

★

My mother taught me to swim.

Chapter 6: Salt as Cure

'I believe you are unhappy, Jonathan,' he said.

'I am unhappy, Father,' I said. 'I have loved this town and the people in it. I have drunk them down with delight. But they have some poison in them which I cannot stand. If I think of them now, I vomit up my soul. Do you know of a cure for me?'

'Why, yes,' he said, 'I know of a cure for everything: salt water.'

'Salt water?' I asked him.

'Yes,' he said, 'in one way or the other. Sweat, or tears, or the salt sea.'

'The Deluge at Norderney' from *Seven Gothic Tales*
by Isak Dinesen (Karen Blixen)

Dozens of 'cures' are touted as treatment for Depression. I know this because I was always on the lookout for them, always on the hunt for ways to mend Mum. Surely, I told myself, *surely* if I looked hard enough, long enough, in the right places, I'd find one. And, just to be certain, just to make sure I didn't miss anything, I set up a Google News Alert – *Depression* – to sift from the ether anything of significance.

Sometimes Google spat out nuggets of meteorologic import, warning of low-pressure weather systems which would deliver wind and rain. Sometimes it pointed me in the direction of economic collapse. And I puzzled: how are we to take an illness seriously when it shares its moniker with words the meteorological department or bankers might use?

When I consider this habit now, when I think about it in the cold light of years of experience, I know it smacks of desperation – why would I find something that worked where my mother's doctors had not? And yet, it is so tempting to imagine there is something hiding in plain sight, *surely if I looked hard enough, long enough, in the right places, I'd find it:* an elixir

When you are desperate you are easily seduced by alchemy peddled as remedy. Snake oil, the journalist John Diamond called it, of the 'cures' touted for his cancer.

There was no cure for my mother's Depression. If there had been, she would not have endured so many years of illness. There were only drugs that mediated it, that made the lows less crippling, the trajectory of her return to health a little steeper. There were pills that tamped down the bright burn of it, blunted its worst edges. Made us feel at least we were doing *something*, at least she was *trying*.

That's the best we got.

But we only understood that after we'd succumbed to the lure of a 'cure'.

*

The nutritionist's clinic was held in her plush home in an expensive quarter of a seaside town. She invited us to take a seat in her large sunny sitting room. Mum, brimming with good health at the time (her 'time to be well'), was all smiles and conversation and excited at whatever miracle this woman might conjure, the wave of a wand and Mum's Depression would vanish forever like a card up a sleeve – the essence of eternal *joie de vivre* in its place.

'Would you like some chamomile tea?' the nutritionist asked.

Mum – who had never drunk chamomile tea except when unpicked by sleeplessness and anxiety and only then because she was being bullied by me ('Come on, Mum, come on, try it,') – said graciously, 'Oh yes, that sounds lovely!'

'We don't drink coffee in this house, I'm afraid,' continued the nutritionist sounding more smug than apologetic as she considered my expression and registered my poorly disguised disappointment.

What? No coffee?

'Great,' I mumble, 'chamomile tea is great.'

I sit beside Mum, after I've swallowed a polite quantity of insipid pee-coloured brew, in the nutritionist's 'treatment room' and I listen to Mum describe her experience of Depression. She is clear in her delivery, her tone steady, she does not hiccup through tears or hesitation. The voice of my Well Mum. (And I would think later: if Depression changed the tone of my mother's voice, replacing clarity with something timid and hard to hear, Dementia stole the language that gave her a voice at all).

The nutritionist, with her expensively highlighted hair and expertly manicured nails, nods and makes encouraging noises and occasionally winces – like when Mum tips her bag of meds onto the desk between us, as if she is revealing a hoard of illicit contraband. A stash of Class A street drugs – not a prescription legally dispensed by Boots the Chemist.

The nutritionist enquires about Mum's diet, which because she is not sick consists of more than tea and digestive biscuits. It describes the choices of one who eats well: porridge and toast for breakfast, soup and cheese for lunch, fish pie and vegetables for supper. She makes a tutting sound with her tongue when Mum mentions the toast ('all that gluten – so bad for you!') and the cheese ('milk is only meant for baby cows'). She is impressed at Mum's on-off (on only when well) Omega 3 habit, 'But that on its own is not enough,' she warns and Mum's eyes grow round.

She begins to fill in forms with comments and ticks. She directs Mum to a set of scales so that she might register her weight. She considers ranks of tubs of vitamins and minerals, all standing to attention on a shelf beside her. (Like Mum, really). She taps each with a glossy talon as she deliberates its merits in Mum's case. She begins to pluck several forth and describes their system-enhancing attributes to Mum who listens intently and comments with the occasional 'Oh really?' And 'Gosh, I never knew that!' Some cleanse livers, some add energy, some aid sleep and settle nerves, some replenish adrenal burnout.

Allegedly.

And somewhere in the shadows, I think I hear John Diamond's cynical chuckle.

★

The nutritionist is a wizard, she casts a spell over Mum who is persuaded she no longer needs conventional medicine. That she ought to bin all her prescription drugs. There. Then. That very day. She tips the lot down the loo as soon as she gets home so that the venlafaxine capsules bleed pink onto the porcelain and the lithium pills sink like ash in the bowl. Mum is the blind who can suddenly see, the deaf whose world was silent and who can now, in that instant, hear music and laughter and voices, the cripple who with the laying on of hands believes she can walk without her cane. She unpacks bags and boxes of every conceivable vitamin and supplement, and arranges tubs of magic on the kitchen table so that she will be prompted to swallow little pills of promise at every meal.

And then we jointly embark on a rigid diet devoid of dairy and wheat. (And coffee, obviously). I nibble a rice cake smeared with something masquerading as butter for breakfast, and wonder why, if she practised what she preached, the nutritionist was so round. Mum eats with considerably more enthusiasm than me, proclaiming cheerfully, 'I feel so *well*!'

When Mum inevitably succumbed to another episode of Depression a few months later – because as she knew, as we all knew, the nature of her particular beast meant the crest of a wave was always followed by its crashing down, ('It's just my time to be sick') – the fact her system was swimming in expensive supplements did nothing to stop her drowning.

And when she got sick this time, she got sicker than she'd ever been. There were no lingering antidepressants to break the fall, no lithium to temper the low, no anti-anxieties to soothe her fretfulness, nothing to help her sleep: she collapsed. Her cane kicked out from beneath her, she fell hard.

I, furious but hopeful she might still have answers, telephoned the nutritionist and asked what, given the assurances she had made to Mum about continued good health, she recommended.

'Mum is sick again, sicker than I've seen her for years,' I told her. 'What now?' I asked.

The nutritionist didn't sound very pleased to hear from me. The daughter, the doubter.

She considered for a moment.

And then she said, 'I've heard coffee enemas might be useful; I hear they are beneficial in the case of cancer.'

But my mum doesn't have cancer, I wanted to scream, she has *Depression*.

I put the phone down. I didn't know whether to laugh or cry.

But I did know where the coffee had gone.

★ ★ ★

Predictably, given the habit I've developed from years and years of chasing down a cure for Mum's mental illness, a news alert for 'Dementia' joins that for 'Depression.' Both announce themselves every morning with a cheerful little ping as they drop into my inbox. One after the other.

Ping.

Ping.

Ping.

But I'm not looking for cures anymore; I know there are none for Mum. Not now. It's too late: I know there's no debridement of those plaques or unknotting of the tangles that have wound their way around her brain and stolen her stories and are suffocating her intellect and stealing her words. I know this.

But I have learned something about the cause and effect of disease and the merits of prophylaxis. You cannot cure Dementia. But you might be able to prevent it: I'm not looking to save Mum anymore; I can't. I'm looking to save myself.

And yet still I find charlatans hawking hollow hope.

'Foods to Reverse Dementia' one website promises. Reverse? Reverse would be to still those sepia storms, undo the damage. And all Mum needs to do is eat walnuts, salmon, turmeric.

A tabloid newspaper tries to sell me a supplement combination that will slash my Dementia risk by 73 per cent. Even though I (desperate and easily seduced) know this is rubbish, I click and read and then I traipse down the virtual aisles at Amazon to see if I can purchase the quackish prescription they recommend. Omega oil for snake oil. Shake a few capsules into your palm, tip your head back, swallow them with a glass of water and tell yourself that's enough: I am safe.

But I am not. It is not that simple. So many things unspool our mind, so much is needed to keep it tightly wound.

'Fucking blueberries,' raged Amy Bloom in her memoir, *In Love*, about her husband's early onset Dementia, 'There is literally no treatment. The most advanced Alzheimer's research in the world says, eat fucking blueberries, get enough fucking sleep.'

Mum didn't get enough of either.

★

The 2020 *Lancet* Commission tells us there are twelve modifiable risk factors for Dementia. Modifiable means things you can do something about to reduce your risk of developing the disease; 40 per cent of cases are influenced by things we can influence. There are the obvious ones: watch your weight, don't smoke, keep an eye on blood pressure, stay active, mind your sugar intake, eat a balanced diet – include blueberries and walnuts if it makes you feel better. Broadly, the message is 'what's good for your heart is good for your head' – the mantra of many doctors including Dr Albert Hofman, chair of the Department of Epidemiology at Harvard T H Chan School of Public Health.

'After all,' he said to me, 'Without a circulation, there is no brain function.'

Hofman and his team revealed rare, encouraging (and given the sometimes snake-oil-selling nature of the internet, credible) news about Dementia. They tracked the health of 50,000 adults over the age of 65 to understand how the risk of Dementia had changed over the past two decades. What they found was that there had been a decline of 13 per cent every ten years from 1988 to 2015. Hofman attributes this to better – and better awareness of – heart health.

About 30 to 40 per cent of all cases of Dementia are related to vascular factors, he says, and in principle these can be – and, as demonstrated by Hofman's work, have been – prevented by attacking vascular risks with things like hypertensives, cholesterol-fighting drugs, better awareness in terms of diet and physical activity and – significantly – the decline in smoking.

It is not just the direct effects of cardio and vascular diseases that negatively impact the brain – it's also the indirect effects of the inflammatory processes that come with heart disease which can have a negative effect, he reminds me.

But one of the biggest challenges, says Hofman, is the public's fatalistic attitude towards Dementia as an inevitable disease of the elderly; we have to change behaviour to avoid it, he says. Because we can.

There has been, says Hofman 'Enormous success in the last part of the last century and the early part of this one in preventing heart attack and stroke' and the same could apply to Dementia. We might not eradicate it, he says, but if we could push it to a later phase in life at least then people would have more years of quality living and may die, he says, 'for want of a better phrase: a better death.'

A better death for a condition that in the decade to 2022 took more lives in Britain than any other illness, more than cancer or heart disease. A doctor tells me, 'People are more afraid of getting Dementia now than they are of Cancer; the Big D is bigger than the Big C.' (And I think, 'So it's not just me that ascribes capitals to illnesses.')

I watch my mother and I know Hofman is right. There are better ways to die.

★ ★ ★

British writer Raynor Winn and her husband Moth lived to walk. But they learned, over the thousands of miles they've marched, that they walked to live. Especially in Moth's case; he was diagnosed with a neurodegenerative disease, corticobasal degeneration, in 2013, the same week the couple were made homeless.

The same week again, armed with tents and wearing walking boots, the couple set out to walk the UK's 630 mile-long South West Coast Path. Not only did it lead to Winn's bestselling book, *The Salt Path*, but it also improved Moth's health. Worried, post pandemic, that Moth was deteriorating, they decided to do it again, but walk bigger, further. This time they walked the length of Britain, one thousand miles. Another book, *Landlines*, followed. And so too did an improvement in Moth's condition.

Winn asked at the end of their walk, 'Can using a body in the way it was made to be used reverse symptoms that are thought to be irreversible?' She doesn't think so. And yet, as they sit in her husband's consultant's office awaiting the result of his latest CT scan, that's exactly what they see: darkness to light.

'What would you like to see?' the consultant asks Moth.

'I'd like to see the screen lit up like a Christmas tree,' says Moth. The consultant turns the screen towards him. Winn is too afraid to look. 'There you have it, there's your Christmas tree,' says the doctor.

'The screen is alight,' observes Winn.

★

Ping: People who walk 3,800 steps a day are about 25 per cent less likely to develop Dementia, a news alert from Harvard Health announces.

A few weeks later: *Ping!* It's not enough to walk further than you might already, you need to walk faster: *Walk Far, Walk Fast to Reduce Dementia Risk*

Fast? How fast is 'fast'? At least 100 paces a minutes. I step mine up to 125. I breathe hard. I feel sweat lick my back.

Why fast walking though? There's the obvious – getting the heart pumping (*what's good for your heart is good for your head*). There's also telomeres. It's down to telomeres, says the science.

Telomeres are the 'caps' at the end of chromosomes. They help protect our DNA just like the plastic tips at the end of shoelaces protect them from unravelling.

I consider the little caps at the end of my laces now, as I tie them tight, ready to walk. I touch them, make sure they are secure, I touch them as you might touch wood. If they pop off, those innocent, ordinary caps, my laces will begin to fray: there, right there: a visual prompt. A reminder.

Walking fast is associated with longer telomeres, which in turn is associated with slower ageing; a lifetime of brisk walking could cut as many as sixteen years off your biological age by midlife.

I have heard this word before – *telomere* from the Greek *telos* 'end' and *meros* 'part'. Once, long ago, and while exploring my mother's Depression, I stumbled upon a paper that found people with major Depression have shorter telomeres; the severity of their condition and duration of episodes was inversely correlated to telomere length. That's why, research says, longer telomeres are a marker of psychological resilience. I check my laces again; I touch the end of those caps. Again.

Was my mother, with her short telomeres, vulnerable to a life of foreshortened independence? And was that because Depression kept her pinned to a chair, in a bed, not a single walk for weeks, months, at a time so that Dementia caught up with her?

It's not just that walking is good for our brains, it's that sitting too long is bad for them.

The negative effects of extended sitting can be so strong, researchers found, that even people who exercise regularly bear a higher risk if they sit for ten, twelve, 15 hours in the day even if they exercised for an hour in between times; Sit for 10 hours and the risk rises 8 per cent, 12 hours and it's 63 per cent, 15 hours and it soars 321 per cent.

321 per cent!

(I begin to pay attention when the little green man on my fitness tracker dances his irritating jig and fizzes impatiently because I've been at my desk too long.)

This is obviously in part because moving improves cardiovascular fitness – *look after your heart*… Less obviously, aerobic exercise, even if not vigorous, increases growth factors in the brain that help preserve existing brain cells and may prompt the growth of new ones.

And third, when we move, our brains aren't just working

to cause that movement and support our balance, they also, as one expert explained to me 'Keep track of where we're going so that we can (hopefully) get back. This doesn't just involve our eyes but also the positions of our joints, our heads, and the sounds around us. The brain works hard to remember all that information. When the brain works hard, new connections—and sometimes new brain cells—are made to enable new memories.'

I get up from my desk more often to walk more steps and I up my pace to 140. It feels like turning my back on something and getting ahead of it as quickly as I can.

'Does it matter how late in life one embarks on a brisk walking programme?' I ask one expert.

'Nope,' he is emphatic, 'It's never too late to start.'

It's only ever too late to turn back.

And I think of Winn's question: 'Is 1,000 miles far enough to turn darkness into light?'

★ ★ ★

I introduce myself to the authors of the most credible research as a journalist with an interest in neurodegenerative disease (to lend some gravitas and professional credibility) and as 'my mother's carer.'

I am shameless.

Carer. The lexicon of kindness. They have to respond: a guilt-tripping tug of heart strings – *look at me, poor me, my poor Mum* – and they can't say no. They'll answer my questions – sometimes they'll even give me airtime on Zoom. They'll grant me access to all the papers I can't access because they're behind a paywall. I will pore over them, uncomprehending of much of the terminology, most of the language, but determined to understand. 'Keep doing hard stuff,' one doctor told me, 'to build your cognitive reserve.' 'Stump yourself' urges the US Alzheimer's Association.

I am evangelical. I am a bore. To my husband: 'How many steps have you done today? What are you reading? What's your waist measurement? What are you going to do when you retire – you can't just stop; your brain will atrophy.'

'Enough,' he says, holding up a hand: 'Enough. Just because your mother has Dementia doesn't mean we're all going to get it.'

'But you don't know the numbers...'

He puts his hand up again, 'I do. You've told me. I do.'

'... somebody in the UK is diagnosed with Dementia every three...'

My husband is an optimist.

And that's a good thing: an optimistic attitude to life may be prophylactic according to something I read in January.

My mother's Depression stole her hope and then it drained her reservoir.

2022 (After)

For a few brief months, my mother was concerned she was pregnant.

(To compute the improbability of this – an 82-year-old who'd had her womb removed forty years earlier – was way beyond Mum's reach: *I'm not nearly that old!* Or, *How would you know if I'd had a hysterectomy anyway?*)

'Look at the size of my tummy,' she would fret, patting it as – come to think of it – an expectant mother might her bump.

I laughed then, 'You're not having a baby, Mum, I just feed you too well!'

She looked doubtful – whether at the lack of my culinary skills or the lack of a pregnancy, I'm unsure.

For a while after she came to live with me, she ate with gusto and, as her waistband began to strain, I was obliged to keep trying to find her bigger and bigger trousers. 'Get a size 14,' I tell my sister, 'Or a 16,' when she sends me the link for a pair of drawstring pants online. Zips are troublesome once you're in diaper-clad Dementia land. They take too long.

We told ourselves, the rounder Mum got, 'At least she enjoys her food.'

At least she enjoys her food. Because it was the last thing she could.

If my slender mother ever put on weight, it was always there, always around her middle.

Was this of significance?

I find a study about abdominal fat as a risk for Dementia; I read that it predisposes a person to brain shrinkage.

Really? It seems so far-fetched, that middle-aged spread might mean a thinning of cognition.

You won't be surprised to know I appeal to the authors of the study:

I'm a journalist with an interest in Dementia. I care for my mother in late-stage AD…

I bombard them with questions: why might abdominal fat make a person susceptible to brain shrinkage? What's the link? Why fat around the middle, specifically? Why not fat around the buttocks or thighs, say?

'Because,' they tell me, 'excess fat increases inflammation and inflammation increases the risk of brain atrophy.' But why the abdomen, I press? 'Because that's the most common site for fat deposition,' they tell me. And, they add, 'Stress and poor sleep encourage visceral fat, that's the type that clings to our internal organs.'

Stress and poor sleep. I puzzle at how Depression could steal my mother's appetite while simultaneously 'ribboning her insides with gleaming yellow,' which is how the researchers describe this sort of fat to me.

Devil's guts; strangle-weed; witch's hair.

They send me MRI images to illustrate the point and even to my untrained eye it is obvious. There it is, in compelling black and white: with the gathering bulk of a person's frame about their midsection, the settling of that fat, so there is the spreading shadow of atrophy in their brain, as if the inside of their heads is being eaten alive.

★ ★ ★

I stand beneath an icy shower and count: *One, two, three.* I need to stand here for a whole minute.

I leap into swimming pools brittle with the cold and emerge with an ice-cream headache.

Can Cold Water Cure Dementia? asks one site.

The next day, Google shares this fact: cold-water swimming may protect the brain from degenerative diseases such as Dementia.

Swimmers who swam at a London lido had their blood analysed and tested positive for a 'cold-shock' protein which scientists found slowed cognitive decline in mice.

Cooling can help to protect brains when they might be vulnerable to damage: people with head injuries, premature babies. Doctors know this. Could the same apply to Dementia? When animals hibernate, they cull brain synapses as a way to slow their systems down and conserve resources. When they come to, after a long wintering, these synapses – the connections that relay messages in our brains, the signalling systems that become unstable and undone in Dementia – unfurl like the fresh, new green of tender spring growth.

People began to leap into frozen lochs in Scotland with reckless abandon so that scientists are forced to urge caution and remind the public that hypothermia comes with a slew of brain-damaging risks as well.

Desperate!

* * *

One day during one of our blind Skype calls, Mum tells me she is reading a book called *Lady Icarus*.

'That's a funny title!'

'It is!' she laughs, 'Set in France, I think.'

She's right: it's the eighteenth-century story of Sophie Blanchard, the first professional female aeronaut who was, indeed, French.

I ask Mum if she has been to France.

The silence on the other end of the line tells me she does not know.

But she has: she went to school there.

How to sensitively fill in your forgetting parent's past using words that do not scream of frailty or madness?

That means I am demented.

'You told me about your French friends at school in Honfleur,' I nudge, 'About Town Annique and Country Annique and how Country Annique's family would bathe once a week, on a Saturday, before they went to play baccarat at the local Casino.'

Something like remembering flits across her face and then it's gone, the sputtering of a lamp when you flick the switch and the bulb fizzes then pops.

I try something different: I say, '*Bonjour Mama, ça va bien*?'

'*Oui*,' she says, '*Oui, je vais très bien, merci*.'

Months after this conversation, over supper one night, Mum remarks, as she peers at the mangetout I have spooned onto her plate 'I thought you were supposed to take peas out of their skins before you cooked them.'

'Try the shells,' I tell her.

She looks at me as if I've asked her to eat potato peelings out of a bin.

'No THANK you!'

'Try them, Ma, they're good; you're *meant* to eat them.'

She daintily peels a shell into thin strips and puts a tiny slice into her mouth.

'Not bad,' she sniffs.

'They're mangetout, Ma. What does that mean?'

'Eat all,' she says, without a second's hesitation.

Google tells me being bilingual could delay symptom-onset of Alzheimer's by an average of five years, making, one website assures me, 'language-learning apps such as Duolingo a superior alternative to pricey new medications.' It elaborates: That's because second-language proficiency matters more than when a language was learned, 'meaning that learning any new language at any age protects against Alzheimer's symptoms.'

The Duolingo app on my phone has been starved by lack of use and is slumped, skin and bone, in a desert:

Revive your learning habit, scolds the skeleton glaring at me accusingly from enormous eye sockets.

Mum went to school in France 65 years ago. She remembers phrases from the language, but not that she was ever there. Is there any point in that: in knowing the words but not the story?

I revive Duolingo with a single ten-minute lesson about oranges and dogs.

If only it were that easy.

* * *

A 2019 survey by Alzheimer's Disease International found that 62 per cent of medics think Dementia is a normal part of ageing. That it's inevitable.

It isn't.

One in four people think there's nothing you can do to avoid it.

But there is.

You can walk fast, frequently, further. You can eat better. You can take blood pressure meds and statins if you need to. You can keep an eye on your sugar. You can read, learn, stretch yourself. You can do hard stuff to fill your cognitive reserve to the brim.

You can get your vision checked.

You can get your hearing tested.

Researchers at Johns Hopkins found that even mild hearing loss doubled the risk of cognitive impairment. Moderate loss tripled that risk, and people with a severe hearing impairment were five times more likely to develop Dementia.

Why? Well, a Senior Research Associate at the Cochlear Center at Johns Hopkins tells me, there are three mechanisms that may explain why hearing loss might be associated with Dementia.

First, and I expect this: hearing loss can make communicating with others more difficult, which can exacerbate social isolation, another of the *Lancet*'s modifiable risk factors for Dementia.

Secondly, when hearing is compromised, 'Speech and sound are garbled by the time they reach the brain, which requires it to use extra effort to process and decipher those sounds. As a result, the brain then has fewer resources for activities like memory and executive function, which can eventually lead to cognitive impairment.'

Thirdly, with hearing loss, the parts of the brain that are stimulated by speech and sound are no longer stimulated, which can lead to atrophy and changes in brain structure and function.

Hearing loss can begin at just 45. Forty per cent of people over fifty have some degree of hearing loss. Loss they mightn't be aware of; changes to our hearing happen very gradually and over time. Hearing loss is silent too, it seems.

With normal hearing, a person can decipher, for example, people breathing, mosquitoes whining, leaves rustling in a breeze. Mild hearing loss may be present if you can't hear the fridge humming or people whispering. If you have moderate hearing loss you mightn't be able to hear rain falling or the bubble and hiss of coffee percolating.

But how bad exactly would hearing loss have to be to impact cognition?

Every 10-decibel increase in hearing loss is associated with 16 per cent greater prevalence of Dementia. An example of a 10 dB difference? Consider that 20dB is whispering from five feet away and 30dB is whispering nearby.

Get a hearing test over fifty, the experts advise me. So I do, to the bafflement of the ENT specialist I consulted.

'But are you actually experiencing hearing difficulties?' No, I confirm, 'But I just want to check.'

I want to check so much I pay for a private consultation with an audiologist who puts me into a soundproof cubicle in a clinic in North London and instructs me to don a pair of headphones and then to register every sound I hear, no matter how faint.

Some of the sounds are very faint. I take no chances. I mark every single sound I think I hear, sifting the slightest one from a background of white noise. I need to pass this test, I tell myself.

And, despite trying my hardest, I am, to my horror, because I thought I heard perfectly well, diagnosed with mild – mild but advanced for my age – hearing loss.

*

Ophthalmologists who studied 3000 older adults found the risk of Dementia was higher among those with vision problems; a third of those with moderate or severe distance impairment had signs of Dementia.

Their findings mirror those of previous studies, including one which found that elderly people who underwent cataract removal surgery had a 30 per cent lower risk of developing Dementia compared with participants who didn't have the surgery.

There are several hypotheses as to why loss of vision might be a risk factor for Dementia.

In some cases, there may be a common neurodegenerative or vascular cause of vision loss and Dementia. Then there's the obvious fact of how compromised vision might lead to a decrease in physical activity and social engagement, both risk factors for Dementia. Losing your sight decreases your participation in cognitively stimulating activities that buffer against cognitive decline, like reading, pulling the plug on your cognitive reserve.

And, just like with hearing, you can test your sight, and not just so you've got the right specs to read, drive, keep working, but because a simple eye test can flag dangerous diagnoses: glaucoma is often referred to as the 'silent thief of sight' because it's asymptomatic.

I make a note to get my eyes checked after my hearing test. I am reminded: We need to remain connected to our world through our senses to make sense of that world.

* * *

There is a photograph of my mother on my desk. In it, she is smiling a wide, white-toothed smile. Her Dementia was evident everywhere in our lives by then – but not in the picture: from the photo you'd never guess. She looks self-possessed and whole. Her hair, after a rare visit to the salon, is neat and closely cropped. She looks straight into the lens. She looks, I think now, with her Colgate smile, like a commercial for geriatric dental care.

I wish she'd always had teeth like that; she was very conscious of her smile when she had her own teeth. Two years before the photo in question was taken, she'd had her top teeth removed, all of them. They were loose and discoloured. Her falsies transformed her face, her smile.

What I never imagined was that her teeth might have been another marker for Dementia later.

Oral health is linked to more than just fillings. Poor oral health is associated with many common diseases:

cardiovascular disease, diabetes, rheumatoid arthritis, even neurodegenerative diseases, like Dementia.

That's because the mouth is connected to important systems – respiratory, digestive, cardiovascular – and contains numerous microorganisms, some of which can harm our health. If we are not vigilant about looking after our teeth, the build-up of plaque creates a breeding ground for bacteria which can lead to gum disease. And those bacteria, if not checked, might travel through our systems, infecting and triggering inflammation in other body tissues, including the brain.

If my grandmother's generation used to say you lost a tooth for every child you bore, in mine, losing a tooth equates to an extra year of brain ageing. Some research suggests people with poor dental hygiene are 21 per cent more likely to develop Alzheimer's disease.

It's not just about blood-brain barrier infections and inflammation, though. Scientists hypothesise that oral bacteria produce an enzyme which interacts with nerve cells in the brain, releasing a protein that leads to cell death. Once the nerve cell dies, the protein attaches itself to healthy neighbouring cells, repeating the process and causing further damage in the brain as the disease spreads.

Not brushing your teeth, (and when she was sick with Depression my mother's self-care went the way of everything: nowhere), not going to the dentist, we know these are bad habits if we want to uphold good oral care. But what about the things that sneak in and undo us? Many antidepressants cause a dry mouth – xerostomia – which can lead to periodontal disease and tooth decay. We need a healthy amount of saliva to maintain a healthy mouth. One dental surgery suggested that 100 per cent of patients suffer consequences from their antidepressant prescription.

And I remember my mother's regular refrain, 'My mouth is as dry as a bone.'

If she didn't have the energy to brush her teeth often enough in Depression, in Dementia she often could not remember how.

I accompany her to the bathroom each evening to help her brush the few teeth she has left in her mouth. Her false teeth smile at us from a glass by the sink.

She picks up her toothbrush and considers it.

'How do I use this? Which end?'

I turn it the right way around. I smear the tiniest bit of paste on the bristles.

'Brush, Ma,' I say.

She starts then stops, 'Am I doing this right?'

I consider my smile in the mirror later as I clean my own teeth. It's not straight or very white. But it is strong. My dentist confirms this with an x-ray – there is no bone loss, no gum disease, but, she says, 'You're brushing far too hard.'

And I cannot be sure whether I do this to keep my teeth or keep my memories.

After

Mum's days are shrinking. So is she. She grows tinier and tinier as her appetite diminishes. The full mugs of tea she used to drink, one after another, are now rare, meagre half cups. Two thick slices of breakfast toast now a thin quarter, often dropped to the dog. Everything about her is getting smaller, even her conversation; the only thing that's getting bigger are the gaps. Gaps in understanding. In reasoning. In her memories.

Her language, too. Words are harder to find. She abbreviates them. Or chops them up. Or they trail off in a frustration of stuttering.

Years ago, Mum remarked as we listened to a storm, 'What makes the thunder? Is there something solid up there? It sounds as if something big is being moved around'.

I had smiled at her fanciful imagination. I did not know it was fate laying the first bricks for those castles in the air.

Today: 'Listen,' she says, as she cocks an ear to the sound of a storm being herded in by crowds of clouds, 'Can you hear the pre-rain noise?'

My heart cracks. I think the noise of it breaking might be louder than the thunder my mother describes.

But later, she is galvanised: 'I must read more,' she tells me as she browses through the pile of books I have placed by her chair. Children's titles mostly. I tell her I do this because the print is bigger and so the words clearer, easier to read with fading sight.

'Thank you,' she smiles, 'That's thoughtful of you.'

A lie. Another lie. I do it in the hope some small part of this childish story will make sense. Entertain. Gift her a glow of something like achievement.

I hold her upright for the shortest walk. She leans into me now. The curve of her spine seems to make her list.

'You're drifting,' I laugh, 'You're just like that ship of yours.'

She laughs. But I don't think she gets the joke.

'I really must walk more,' she says and slows to a halt. Her breathing is hard. Her top lip is dewed by beads of sweat with the effort of all this.

'I just must do more.'

I don't ask, 'Do more what?'

'Yes,' she says again, as if to say it twice will summon it to stick, 'I must do more.'

She makes this promise with such conviction, a vigour that belies her frailty. When she was sick with Depression, we begged her to try to do more, to do better, tomorrow.

She sighed then and said, 'I'll try. But I can't promise.'

Now my vanishing mother pledges: 'I will. I will start tomorrow.'

'Excellent, Mum. You must,' I say, 'Walking is so good for us, it keeps us going, walk more before it's too late and you can't walk at all.'

And with that, Mum steps up her pace as if to prove to me she means what she says.

* * *

'It's not easy to avoid Dementia,' a doctor tells me, 'And it's hard to look at health long-term,' he adds, nervous of my evangelist enthusiasm, 'especially when we are still relatively young and completely well.' There is, he warns, a large element of fate.

But, he concedes, because he cannot resist my pressing optimism, 'There is a great deal you can do to protect yourself.' It's why the *Lancet* urges us to be 'ambitious' about preventing Dementia. Fending off this disease calls for a robust armour. A handful of Omega 3s with your breakfast isn't enough. Really. You need to rally the troops.

All the troops.

*

Months after I first stumble across his storm warning of a 'silent tsunami' – *We talk about there being a long, silent period of this disease before Dementia develops, but it's only silent because we are not listening properly* – I ask Craig Ritchie *how* we could listen better.

I feel something like vindication when he tells me it's not just the likes of me – daughters who sense the undercurrent tug of change manifesting in their mothers too late – it's clinicians too. Many don't just fail to hear it; they don't believe there's any way to change its course.

There's an 'endemic nihilism,' he says, among the medical community, 'that there's nothing we can do about this illness.' The problem is, he says, 'we're dealing with the legacy of the twentieth century': *Senile Dementia.*

Senile – derived from the French *sénile* or Latin *senilis,* whose roots grew from *senex,* for 'old man'. The very word suggests it's an unavoidable part of ageing – and we all get old. Is it that resignation to a fate described by language that stalls the science? Or is it because if we're near the end of our lives anyway, our lives don't count? That the science isn't worth chasing?

Except it is. The brain changes that undo a person in their seventies or eighties – when they lose their way, forget their history, can't remember their daughters – manifest much earlier in life, in our fifties and sixties.

Its tiny seeds germinate and thread a scrawny root meanly in thin soil to anchor a skinny seedling, then the plant begins to grow – greedily – in the direction of a host.

'If we could detect Alzheimer's before it spreads, then I believe we can cure it within ten years,' says Ritchie.

Detect it? How? Blood tests to measure biomarkers, the pointers to this illness: amyloid, the protein that settles as plaque in the brain, amyloid which triggers the toxic neurofibrillary tangles of tau that tie our thinking into knots then pull it all apart in our unravelling. Memory clinics which might flag – earlier – slowing cognition so that lifestyle risk could be measured in numbers: How much do you weigh, how much do you smoke, how much do you drink, what's your blood pressure, how many steps do you walk each day? Count the numbers and you can begin to calculate – and then subtract – the risks: vascular, diabetes, 'inflammageing'.

We need to treat Alzheimer's Disease – both with medicine and attitude – much earlier, says Ritchie. We need to treat it before, or even as, amyloid is cementing itself as plaque between neurons and beginning to interrupt our intricate messaging systems. We need to have faith in the drugs that clear amyloid from the brain, says Ritchie, the faith to harness their power before the illness reveals itself in characteristic symptoms.

I listen to a neurologist being interviewed on the radio in response to the licensing of a new Alzheimer's drug. He is scathing of these new medicines – their side effects are too great, he warns. I listen to him and I can't help wondering if he has ever loved – and lost – somebody (again and again and again) to this death-by-a-thousand-cuts disease? If my mother had had the choice between losing herself or taking the risks that come with this early – yes, experimental – medicine, what would she have opted for? What would you choose?

And anyway, he continues, the attendant financial costs of developing these drugs are too great.

In 2019, the annual global societal costs of Dementia were estimated at over $1.3 trillion. Will the costs of developing the right drugs ever exceed that? In 2020, the cost of bringing a new drug to market was between $300 million and $3 billion.

Besides, he adds, their intravenous administration is too time-consuming. But will they gift back the hours lost in caring? Has he read *The 36-Hour Day: A Family Guide to Caring for People Who Have Alzheimer Disease and Other Dementias*? Will the slow drip-drip of drugs into a person's system over a few days each month protect them from years lost in autonomy? Will it keep all the words of all their stories printed on the page so that nothing fades to illegibility?

It would be unthinkable, as Ritchie says, for an oncologist to discover a malignant lump in a woman's breast and send her away with a terminal prognosis. An oncologist will do everything to eradicate a tumour *in situ* before it metastasizes. And even after it has, the arsenal that fights cancer is loaded and loaded again and aimed and fired: chemotherapy, radiotherapy, immunotherapy, more surgery to whichever organ the malignancy has spread.

Yet the brain, the organ that directs, orchestrates, choreographs the healthy functioning of every other organ in the body? We will leave that to its plaque-and-tangled fate?

HIV/AIDS is the other analogy Ritchie uses to demonstrate the speed at which medicine can advance when it must.

Gay-Related Immune Deficiency (GRID) – as it was initially called – was first diagnosed in 1981. It was renamed Acquired Immune Deficiency Syndrome (AIDS) in 1982. The WHO launched a global surveillance in 1983. In 1985, the first commercial blood test for HIV was licensed by the FDA.

The same year, the CDC (Centers for Disease Control and Prevention) reported an 89 per cent increase in AIDS diagnoses in a year. It predicted the number would double in 1986. By that year, the first anti-retroviral drug, AZT, was available.

Within a decade of this terrible disease revealing itself, HIV/AIDS had a name, a test, a treatment.

By 1996 the number of AIDS cases diagnosed every year in the States began to decline; the illness ceased to be the leading cause of death for Americans between their mid-twenties and mid-forties.

Today, 1 in 9 people aged 65 and older in the States has Alzheimer's. Coincidentally, in the USA, at the peak of the AIDS pandemic, one gay man in nine had been diagnosed with the disease.

In 2020, Alzheimer's Disease International reported that there were 55 million people in the world living with Dementia. This number, they warned, will double every twenty years.

What drove the urgency then, with AIDS? Was it because a younger generation could campaign energetically – and they did, for themselves, their lovers, their brothers, their sons – for awareness, recognition, better care? What stalls the medical community now? Is it because we don't hear the old people with Dementia? Don't see them? Because they don't have a voice?

I think about the 'nihilism' Ritchie refers to; a collective shrug in the face of something we deem par for the course, *senile Dementia*, the inevitable consequence of old age.

Ten years, Ritchie said.

'If we could detect Alzheimer's before it spreads, then I believe we can cure it within ten years.'

Chapter 7: Adrift

In his book, *Why We Remember*, neuroscientist Charan Ranganath describes memory's most important feature as not 'replaying the past but orienting us to the future.'

Our memories, he says, 'enable us to allocate critical resources to what is new and what has changed.'

When I am forty, Anthony accepts a job in a very remote corner of western Tanzania. There are no asphalt roads into the place. Nor – more importantly – out of it. It takes two hours to fly in from the capital city. The plane hangs above bush threaded with the dusty ribbons of cattle-tread, and I only know we are drawing close to civilisation, just before we touch down, when a small tin-roofed settlement erupts like silver foil smeared over scrub.

I had not wanted to be here.

'You don't have to come with me,' said my husband, aware of my resistance, 'But I'd like it if you did.'

Conflicted, as I tried to decide what was best, for me, for him, for our family, I made lists. 'Pros' and 'Cons'; 'Here' or 'There'.

'Would you go?' I asked my girlfriends.

'What! There? No fear,' they said, 'Are you mad?'

I asked my son, my daughters: Would two homes be okay? Us here, near school. Dad there. For work.

'Nope.' They were adamant: 'We want one home, with you *and* Dad in it.'

And then I asked Mum: 'What would you do?'

Mum, who used to say, whenever we were faced with a difficult choice, 'You can have one or the other, not both, pick one,' didn't have to think about it. 'Yes,' she said, 'I'd go.' And I could tell by her tone that she was shocked I'd had to ask.

I had a husband who I had a choice to be with. She didn't.

You can have one or the other, not both. Pick one.

So, I told my husband, 'I'll join you.'

★

It was strange to feel at sea in a landlocked corner of Africa, a forgotten outpost miles from anywhere and *hundreds* of miles from the ocean; I felt adrift.

But what was stranger was finding myself in the dislocated bit of Tanzania my grandmother had once found herself in.

In the late 1940s, in a world lean after two World Wars, when bread was still being rationed in England, and with a global shortage of fats, the British government embarked on a project to redress the shortfall in supply of commodities. They decided to grow peanuts, for the oil, in faraway Tanganyika – as it was then – in Africa, a place synonymous with savers and slavers: David Livingstone and Tippu Tip.

The Groundnut Scheme was carved into land where the soil was mostly impenetrable and the landscape, described by the explorer, Henry Morton Stanley, who first met Livingstone not far from here, blanketed by 'an interminable jungle of thornbushes.'

Mum, when she still could, recounted the scant recollections of the eight-year-old she was when she got here; she told me about those thornbushes, the 'wait-a-bits'; armed with clutching barbs that would catch your clothes and skin and hair. When you struggled to escape, the thorns would hook you more sharply.

Wait a bit!

She remembered the bees that erupted in angry clouds from that interminable jungle as bulldozers tried to sweep it aside. She remembered their furious swarming as they rose into the air so that from a distance they looked like a pall of smoke. She remembered the storms that would shred the sky with forks of lightning.

But my grandmother, whose memories were never dimmed by Dementia, remembered it all. My growing-up was rich with stories about an India shrugging off the Raj, then Africa slipping the yoke of an empire so that its pink stain on the world began to shrink, like a receding blush of shame.

The places she described, were, to my young ears, the colourful characters of a play: Ootacamund, an Indian hill station, was pretty and self-effacing. Bombay was flamboyant, clamouring for attention, she wore a red bindi on her forehead, a gold ring in her nose. Bangalore was full of mystery. Nachingwea, in Tanganyika's steamy south, was sullen and sea-level hot. Urambo, down the road from where I found myself, was where the groundnuts failed and where lawns were baked to biscuits.

Those places bore the magic of fiction. What I did not know, or did not understand, my childish imagination made up for.

A memory, Ranganath has also said, is not only formed of the things we saw and heard; it's also shaped by our thoughts and our feelings. When you remember something, it's not just about what happened. It's about our interpretation of what happened.

To find myself where my maternal grandmother had been, where her stories lived and breathed, was as if I were reading an epilogue, or studying a map. The memories of those that come before us are the milestones by which we find our way. I know my children have navigated paths because of the memories I have shared. I watched Mum grow quite lost without hers.

My grandmother's outpost of the Fifties was the same and different to mine six decades later. The mango trees were still there, tall sentinel green in tidy ranks of fat shade. The façades of old buildings were grey and pocked with age and the elements. But they were there. Those storms. That sun. They were all still here; I could orient myself by them when I felt lost or lonely.

* * *

Writer and clergyman Robert Burton published his *Anatomy of Melancholy* in 1621. Four centuries later and it still has a place in discussions on mental illness. An Oxford scholar – who took a decade to complete his studies because he was beset so often by his own demons – Burton cited over 13,000 references to capture cause and effect of this malady.

By its sixth edition, at half a million words, it was a doorstop of a book which influenced many literary greats – Milton, Keats, Eliot, Woolf, Beckett. The writer Samuel Johnson wrote that it was Burton's book that got him up and out of bed in the morning.

Burton believed loss was a precursor to melancholy. And I remember Mum's words as I read his, as if the weight of words through history have heaped upon one another to anchor this ancient disease in such similar articulation.

But Burton believed solitude was just as dangerous; he warned that it made a person inclined towards sluggishness, mental agitation. Retreating from the world, he wrote, works 'like a Siren': the mind withdraws so that a person does little but 'ruminate of nothing but harsh and distasteful subjects.'

And I think then of all the weeks and months when we lost Mum to this, to her relentless, useless chewing over the same anxieties. Old worries resurrected as new ghosts with every episode of Depression to haunt her all over again.

As salve to this anguish, Burton advocated occupation: 'I write of melancholy, by being busy to avoid melancholy. There is no greater cause of melancholy than idleness, no better cure than business.'

'Be not solitary, be not idle,' he urged.

I don't remember where, or when, I first encountered his caution. It was years ago. I dig through old correspondence now to see if I can excavate the first reference in my writing.

There. An email to Mum: 'Solitary or idle: One or the other, Mum, one or the other. You can't be both.'

Pick one.

⋆

I repeated the 'solitary or idle' mantra to myself often in my outpost. If the stories my grandmother had shared of her experience here served to signpost a way out of what felt like a void, an hiatus, it was Burton's words that kept me going while I was there.

If I couldn't do anything about the 'solitary' – I was here, wasn't I? – I could do something about the 'idle'. I wrote. I blogged. I interviewed people all over the world for articles, escaping to the four corners of the earth on the magic carpet afforded by the internet.

And if Burton taught me that being lonely was a risk for melancholy, it was from the scholars I found via Google much later that I learned solitary also leaves brains wide open to Dementia, giving those roots the space to grow.

- *Socially isolated older adults have a 27 per cent higher chance of developing Dementia than adults who are socially active.*
- *A Dutch study finds that those who suffer from loneliness have a 64 per cent great risk of suffering cognitive decline.*
- *Loneliness in Elderly Tied to Brain Volume Reduction*

★

Dr Andrew Sommerlad, Associate Professor at University College London's Division of Psychiatry, published a study on the relationship between social participation and Dementia risk which found that greater social involvement in mid and late life was associated with a 50 per cent lower risk for Dementia later.

'Why,' I asked him: 'Why is a social life so good for our brains?'

'Because,' he told me, as his face swam through seas of ether and into my screen, 'social engagement bears a multi-pronged benefit. The elements of stimulation are there in abundance as we put names to faces and remember a person's history, so we can ask about their work or their children. And to captivate an audience with a story means a million neurons must flare simultaneously, to get the joke and laugh in the right places, we need to make important connections.'

'There's a lot going on at once,' he said: 'laughing, talking, arguing, asking questions, remembering the context of a story, discussing what's in the news.' The frivolity of a dinner party – when all the small talk, the frippery, can seem of little consequence when you are able and engaged – is, in fact, an important, textured, multi-layered puzzle. Social interaction boosts our mood – and tamps down the inflammatory effects of cortisol – but it also sharpens our cognition and keeps the circuitry of the motherboard firing in synchronicity.

I think of what my mother was like once. When well, she engaged with curiosity, her expression animated, interested, her focus sharp as she leant towards whomever she was talking to, waiting to prompt with her questions.

When Dementia began to settle into the spaces in her brain, spaces gouged wide by Depression and inoccupation and social dislocation, a disorientated expression would flit across her face mid conversation, like a cloud blotting out the sun.

When she was no longer able to improvise with the little tricks she conjured to paper over the cracks – 'How's the weather in your neck of the woods? Where's that hubby of yours? You'll have to excuse me – my memory isn't what it used to be,' – when she was at sea, she looked stricken.

And she began to ask the same questions over and over and over again: 'Where am I? Who are you? Am I on a ship?'

She lost her skill to ask the incisive questions she'd once asked. Even the questions she managed were no good to her; she never remembered the answers.

* * *

If my grandmother was ever overwhelmed by her geography, I never knew, she never said. Had she sifted through her memories and taken only the best bits as keepsakes, left the dull or sharp-edged behind? Had she forgotten? Had I, rapt at her stories, joined the dots up all wrong, coloured between the lines too brightly?

It didn't matter. All that did, now, was that she had survived, even thrived. That her stoicism sustained even if she felt as isolated as I did, was a useful yardstick: If she could do it, so could I.

At least I had Skype.

*

And here, high on dry land, I find it is swimming that helps to keep me afloat again. I *make* myself swim at dawn.

I plough up and down the pool and watch a fat sun heave itself up over a horizon that is being drawn in by the dawn so I can see rocky outcrops take shape. I watch it roll into a pale duck-egg blue sky that it will scorch to white-hot by breakfast time. I notice it ignite the tops of the trees in the garden; trees that are beginning to stretch tiny fingerlings of new green, trees that are on fire with flamboyant blossom, bougainvillea that is littering violet blooms.

I begin to *make* myself notice things. Not because I'm making time to stop and smell the roses (I have all the time in the world) but because noticing fills my long days.

I marvel at the water scorpions that scud the surface in quick bursts. I see the day's first brightly coloured lizards creep out of cracks in the wall to seek warmth. They find it in a puddle of sunlight and doze there for a bit. Later, when that side of the house is thrown into shadow and they grow cold, they will scuttle down and lie on the paving stones which by then will be too hot for me to walk across in my bare feet. I have studied their sunbathing habits; seen how they tolerate the scalding stone for so long. I have watched how they do this: resting their weight on their heels while they raise their toes and their tails, so that the most sensitive parts of their bodies aren't burned on sun-baked cement.

★ ★ ★

Scientists who study how being busy supports healthy brain function have found that the busier a person is, the better their memory. It is no coincidence that verbal memory declines 38 per cent faster after retirement. Nor, then, is it surprising that David Merrill at Pacific Brain Health told me he thinks 'pursuit' is a better word than 'hobby', for it speaks to the urgency of maintaining an active, engaged lifestyle.

In keeping busy you are constantly maintaining cognition, as if in the planning of a task, its execution, moving onto the next, you are a flame to the tangle of neurons in your head, lighting them so that they flare bright, are hot with energy and purpose.

For it is not just the doing that is important, it is the fuel of motivation, the after-burn of achievement, that are good for brains: a sense of purpose is associated with a 19 per cent reduced rate of clinically significant cognitive impairment.

The opposite of purpose is apathy, a significant part of Dementia.

And a symptom of every one of my mother's Depressions.

I am inert.

In my outpost, time spilled like the sky and the views and the space, too much of all of it, so much of it that it overflowed. Sometimes I thought I might drown. It was urgency that consumed me then – a hobby would not have carried the necessary ballast, would not have iron-cast my days with direction. It was urgency that punctuated my days so that I knew how to start and when it was okay to stop. It was urgency that compelled me, drove me to stuff those long, loose hours full of something of substance, to weight them with industry, any industry, to make them count. To make *me* count. If time gives definition to our day, it is the use of that time that defines us.

No, filling outpost time was not a hobby.

It was the pursuit of surviving a solitary life.

★

Seven years after I arrived in the place my grandmother once lived, I am packing up to leave. Some of the glass I wrap in tissue paper was hers; it has been here before, too.

I look out at the bougainvillea I pruned and tended to encourage it to flower. Its blossoms skitter across the garden with each exhalation of a breeze, and gather in colourful piles against the fence, like confetti after a wedding that has been and gone.

Chapter 8: Charting New Depths

August 2015 (Before)

When my brother calls, he says, 'Mum's had a stroke. It's nothing to worry about. She's fine.'

I don't know if he says that to manage my anxiety.

Or because the damage had not made its presence felt in lost movement or slowed speech; neither hand was rendered useless by paralysis, he assured me, she was not dragging a foot. She continued to enunciate her words clearly. She could swallow without choking.

She's fine.

We couldn't see it. The broken bit. So until later, we didn't know it was there. Like all the things that have undone Mum, that was disguised too: it snuck in on tiptoes, a masked robber.

And now, now that I know what came afterwards, I will wonder what the fingertip-push on the ranks of dominoes was: my mother's Depression? Or her stroke? Dominoes all standing upright to attention: a nudge, and the first leans forward precariously, then tips itself towards the one in front of it and that tips to the next and the next and the next and before you know it, the whole line has caved in and lies flat.

I will ask her doctor later: 'Why did she have a stroke?'

She did not suffer with any of the usual suspect risks: no high blood pressure or heart disease, no diabetes, a normal cholesterol level. These metabolic risks account for more than 70 per cent of the 15 million strokes that happen globally each year. She did not smoke. She was slender. Her heart beat an even, steady rhythm, no arrhythmia to slow the flow of blood to stagnating pools

So why did she have a stroke? And I am aware, even as I ask my question, that my tone speaks of accusation, as if the diagnosis and the cause are the neurologist's fault. As if I can undermine his words because my mother's many tests have proven her vascular health robust.

He does not miss a beat: 'Because of Depression.'

I must look confused because he elaborates: 'She sat too still for too long. A clot formed: there.'

And he points at my mother's brain scan to show the darkened smudge of damage. 'There? See?'

There it is: that fingertip on a neat column of dominoes.

Depression. Stroke. Dementia. And Mum came tumbling down.

⋆ ⋆ ⋆

Stroke. Say the word. Can you hear a caress in its onomatopoeic delivery? Now say 'struck'. Do you hear the difference? I hear a smack. The crack of a whip.

I do not think the words – *stroke, struck* – are well matched, yet they derive from the same place. 'Stroke' is related to the Greek 'apoplexia' – to rupture, a deadly blow, described, on many of the stroke sites I read later as appearing 'out of the blue'.

A stroke often occurs ***out of the blue****.*

Look for these symptoms that come on suddenly and ***out of the blue****.*

Stroke symptoms generally appear suddenly, seemingly ***out of the blue****.*

Out of the blue. Prophetic as it turned out in Mum's case: a colour for a mood, from the habit of ancient mariners to mark their grief when men died at sea, a banner of blue flags strung above the deck so that their loss would be there for all to see.

That 'out of the blueness' – the Cambridge dictionary defines the phrase as exactly that, *If something happens out of the blue, it is completely unexpected: one day, out of the blue, she announced that she was leaving* – should describe a rarity. *Completely unexpected.* But strokes are not rare: the Centre for Disease Control website tells me that somebody in the States has a stroke every 40 seconds. Every 3 minutes and 14 seconds, someone dies of a stroke. So strokes – given what we know, the numbers we've collated – *should* be better anticipated:

One in four people will have a stroke in their lifetime.

Tsunamis don't happen *out of the blue,* even if you think they do; there's a barely audible shift before they hit; it's how birds know they're coming. Just before the Indian Ocean tsunami struck on Boxing Day in 2004, eyewitnesses noticed birds behaving strangely. Tsunamis produce something called infrasound, a sound with such low frequency, the human ear cannot detect it. Infrasound, like all sound, travels much faster than waves of water. It's how birds, with their super-keen sense of hearing, can detect what's coming and from where long before we notice a thing; they're *listening.*

★

Many doctors don't like the word – stroke. They describe it as being too vague; they'd rather identify what sort of vascular accident happened, and where.

A cerebrovascular injury; an infarct in the left occipital lobe, say. To pinpoint precisely where my mother's brain is struck and where the injury, *out of the blue*, turns healthy brain tissue black so that it dies.

An indelible bruise.

When my brother calls to tell me Mum has had a stroke, it feels like a slap.

Later, much later, when I'm peering down the barrel of Dementia and counting the rounds in the chamber, wondering which I can get rid of to stand a better chance of saving myself, I will learn that one out of every four strokes leads to Dementia.

* * *

There is something familiar about the journey I take afterwards, after my brother's late-night call. An intercontinental flight, overnight, when I am briefly suspended above my world and swaddled by sky and a velvety night so that all I can see is the aircraft's blinking wing light and a waxing moon that slides in and out of my view, keeping pace with me. And all I can hear is the deep resonant hum of jet engines. Time is arrested as I slide north and west and in that hiatus there is something like respite. I am not of any world up here.

This flight reminds me of another, long ago; it reminds me of the intercontinental overnight flight Mum and I took 30 years earlier after Dad's death. There was a peculiar sort of pause then too, as we hung between two lives. A familiar past and a future whose shape we didn't know yet.

I do not know what I will find when I get to where I am going, but in these twelve hours I am at hypnotic remove. It is only when we land, as we bump down onto Dublin airport's runway, that I am jolted out of whatever numbing reverie had offered brief reprieve.

⋆ ⋆ ⋆

I see Mum from across the ward of the brain injury unit, where she has been admitted, before she sees me. She is being supported by two nurses. They are helping her into a jacket.

She turns to watch me as I walk towards her bed and in that instant she is slack jawed, her expression clouded by bewilderment, her mouth open. She looks, for a moment, as if she will not know me. She looks, fleetingly, damaged. And I feel fear bloom.

But then, 'What are *you* doing here?' she asks and I am encouraged by the curiosity, relieved at the clarity of her tone; her words are not smeared by a slur.

I don't answer. I can't. My own words are a knot in my throat which may unravel to tears if I try to tease them out as sentences.

'She's here to see you,' says one of the nurses, 'she's come all the way to see ***you***,' and she smiles at Mum, 'all the way from *Africa*,' and she emphasises the last word, as if to deliver its import, to stress the distance.

'I came as soon as I could,' I say.

March 2015

Six months earlier, and 15 months into the most protracted episode of Depression Mum had ever suffered, I – concerned that she wasn't getting better – travel to England to see for myself why recovery is so resistant this time.

I am appalled at her appearance: She is so thin she has to pin her trousers about her waist or they slip over her hips. And her demeanour is one of complete disinterest – as if she might detach herself and disappear, a child letting go of a balloon. She seems so insubstantial, so reduced by everything Depression has shaved from her, I wonder she has not been spirited away on the wind.

I take her to see a consultant psychiatrist in central London. Mum's voice is lost to her illness. I must speak for her. The consultant asks: 'So how many of these prolonged episodes of Depression have there been since they began? Three? Four?'

Mum gasps. We both stare at him – as if he's said something outrageous, or funny; I almost burst out laughing: 'Oh no,' I say, 'Much more than that, much, much more than that.'

'Yes,' Mum whispers, 'Dozens. Dozens.'

Six days before Mum's stroke, and with her Depression deepening, I wrote to the same consultant again. *She has got much worse,* I say, *she is not getting up, she continues to lose weight, she is not communicating with me, I think a hospital admission might be the only option.*

He responded with a recommendation for – yes – inpatient care. And electroconvulsive therapy, he adds.

That night a clot forms in Mum's brain and lodges itself right at the back, in the bit just above where her head curves elegantly to meet her neck.

It's me who is shocked when I hear she has been rushed to hospital.

★ ★ ★

I wonder, in the seconds it takes me to make three strides across the ward to hug my mother, whether the interior blow to her brain was too big to give Depression the space to stay. *Out! Out! Shoo!* Was it so violent it delivered the necessary force to oust this resistant thing? Would it take up all the space so there wasn't a corner in the blackness to colour in blue? Because Mum looks happy! *Happy.* Happier than I have seen her look in years! Her mouth widens into a smile with hopeful symmetry, there is no palsy here, no droop or drop. And I am relieved to see recognition flood her features.

'How lovely to see you,' she laughs as I wrap her in a hug and feel her smallness against me, like a bird, as if I squeeze too hard she may snap, the top of her head below my chin.

She smells of Johnson and Johnson's baby talc and her hair is scented with a recent shampoo.

★ ★ ★

My mother's stroke – as I explain in a letter to friends later which I tap out as I sit hunched over endless cups of tea in the hospital coffee shop – happened in the left occipital lobe of her brain, 'the back bit, the bit that's responsible for interpreting what a person sees,' I explain. I must comprehend a new lexicon as I navigate the spaces in Mum's brain, get my bearings in this change. This cerebral language. I have done it before – with Depression. We rolled that word around our mouths as something foreign to begin with. Then we used it as often as we could so that it no longer felt like an alien.

Being a left-sided brain injury, Mum's stroke compromises right sided function, causes, in her case, a condition called hemianopia, right-sided blindness. I try to imagine what Mum might see now by holding an open hand over my right eye, a pirate's patch fashioned of my flattened palm. Her occupational therapist tries to describe this to me in a session with her iPad, using an app that simulates what my mother can see.

But I still don't understand the full effect of Mum's vision loss until my sister, who joins me days later, and I conduct an experiment of our own away from the nurses' watchful gaze. We want to understand for ourselves what Mum can and, especially, what she cannot see.

We escort her to a sunlit room at the top of the hospital where it is quiet, where we are confident there will be no interruptions. We instruct Mum to stand in the middle of this bright room. My sister walks towards her from her right side, I from her left. Mum follows my passage without difficulty. She does not know my sister is walking towards her until we meet in the middle:

Then, 'There you are!' she says to my sister with a laugh, 'I thought you'd vanished!'

★

We are at first awkward in our assistance of Mum in rehab. The environment in foreign. Her condition unfamiliar. And Mum, unaware of her new limitations, is not always receptive to our fussing around her; we are all clumsy in attempts to navigate new paths. Mum does not, to begin with, understand she is blindsided so she does not understand why we glue ourselves to her right side as buffers to bruises and collisions with hospital orderlies and nurses and patients in wheelchairs. We are graceless in our attempts to steer her to begin with; we do it too obviously. I am relieved when a nurse shows us, 'See darlings,' she says, 'guide her by her right elbow.' And I notice how she does this, with a subtlety that would suggest Mum is not handicapped. We are just walking in companionable closeness now. We stop the obvious steering and instead behave as tugs along hospital hallways, adjusting our own position in relation to Mum when she veers off course.

'That way,' says Niamh, the kind nurse, 'she won't walk into obstacles she can't see, and you will protect her from people whom she cannot dodge because they don't know she hasn't seen them.'

We practise then, Mum, my sister and I, we walk corridors which ring with the hum of this hospital of the broken-brained. We walk flights of stairs, Mum's right hand on the banisters, me a step behind lest she tip backwards, my sister a step ahead, talking Mum up the stairs as we go, 'Almost there, Mum!' Carol is the bow, and I am the stern. We teach our brother when he visits so that sometimes all three of us surround her like outriggers, trying to protect her from impact and embarrassment. We move through the hospital safely then, a little, laughing flotilla.

Friends and family observe, when they visit Mum in her bright, generous ward with its huge windows and high ceilings, 'You're lucky you got her in here.' Donnybrook, a handsome Georgian building in a leafy part of the city, stands proud within grounds that wrap around it.

It was an eighteenth-century exercise in altruism: the *Hospital for the Incurables.*

I don't know yet that Mum won't be cured. I do not know yet that the cracks we imagine will close over won't, that they will, even with the most solicitous care, widen to great swallowing crevices. I don't know any of that then. It's just as well; if we'd known, we might never have tried as hard as we did.

Every day, for weeks, as September relaxes into autumn, I drive into the city to spend my days with Mum. Dublin is enjoying the flare of an Indian summer, trees aren't sure what to do with themselves and shake their turning heads in confusion. Forty shades of green are softly warming to myriad shades of mellowness; the Virginia creeper that clings to and clambers up dozens of the city's elegant buildings morphs at one end from saffron yellow to turmeric orange to chilli red at the other. Each day that I drive through the city wallowing in a kaleidoscope of mid-season tones, I notice its coat of many colours has changed again: the green is less acid, leaves blush at unexpected, extended warmth and then drop a curtsey and fall to the ground.

More and more, as Mum grows stronger and gains confidence, as she begins, as the doctors promised us she would, to instinctively compensate for her lost vision, we venture into the hospital gardens to walk and Mum remarks upon plants she recognises.

'I know what that plant is,' she says, 'but I don't remember its name.'

I feel a shiver of something unsettling, of something nearly missed or almost lost, the brief cold-water sensation of dread. I can't name the feeling just like Mum – with her passion for garden centres and a library of horticultural tomes – can't name the Butterfly Mint. Or Bergamot. Or the Asters. Or – and this is especially odd – the Dahlias – even though my grandmother planted them in every garden she ever lived in, for their big colourful heads which nodded agreeably.

All the women on Mum's six-bed ward are women of her age who have suffered a similar 'cerebrovascular accident'. Mum gestures to the lady in the bed next to her, who cannot speak or walk, 'I feel so sorry for that lady, whose name I cannot remember.' And I gaze at Mum, stoic, outward looking, courteous, kind and I think, 'This is my Well Mum. My Sick-Well Mum.'

Each ward occupant has a name card above their bed. And Mum, I realise with slow horror, isn't just unable to recall their names, even though she eats three meals a day with these women around a small table set within the ward, she can't read the name cards above their beds either. Is it because she cannot see them? I wonder and I position her so that her sighted side is inclined towards them.

I ask her neurologist, (and I can almost hear his impatient sigh, *not another question*), 'Why is she battling to read? Is that because of the hemianopia?'

No, he tells me, her inability to read has nothing to do with her shrunken vision. It is because the injury has blown a hole in the bit of her brain that correlates to language and reading.

She has developed pure alexia, he pronounces: 'The brain-eye link is broken,' he adds by way of cursory explanation.

And then, because I look uncomprehending: 'She won't be able to read again.'

And I feel another slap.

'Ever?' I ask. Surely, *surely* not, I think.

'Ever?' Mum says in a small voice, looking up from her bed like a child might as her parents discuss her prognosis above her head.

'Ever.'

I do not want to believe this doctor and I especially don't want Mum – who looks appalled – to believe him either, 'He's talking rubbish, Mum' I say, as the doctor stalks off the ward, 'Of *course* you'll be able to read again.'

★

Words on a page are – were – my mother's default: she picks up the written word wherever she finds it, often unthinking, a reflex: a pamphlet in the dentist's surgery, a newspaper in a hotel lobby, a menu in a cafe even when we're only there for a cup of tea.

And words, books, have always been Mum's salvation, especially in the nadir of a Depression. She was able to step into somebody's else's story when her own became too difficult to live in, as if slipping through the backdoor of a wardrobe into some alternative Narnia. Sometimes I thought books were all that were between her and rock bottom; they were a cushion to the worst of it.

And reading has been a mainstay in my life for as long as I can remember. As children, my siblings and I bookended Mum as we sank deep into a sofa on the veranda: my brother with a thumb plugged into his mouth tucked himself beneath one of her arms. I, winding strands of hair about my fingers, leant in on her other shoulder, my sister as a toddler on her lap, and thus bound, we explored the make-believe worlds of *Serafina the Giraffe* and *Babar the Elephant*.

And from reading to us, Mum taught us to read to her. Her finger under each letter as we built words phonetically. She taught us to break them down and sound them out and put them back together again, bit by bit. As if slotting the pieces of a jigsaw together and finding that they fit neatly to make something we could recognise. Cat. Dog. Red. And then, like magic, the letters made words which delivered a story that I could see reflected in the picture I saw.

Later, much later, Mum taught me to teach my own children to read. My bookshelves sag with the weight of books she gifted me, sent to her grandchildren, books that she chose with care from a catalogue she examined with morning tea, a pen poised as she circled the titles she thought they might like. And I read to my own children as she read to us, three circled around me vying to be closest, bickering when they couldn't see the page, a head tucked under my arm, small plump fingers curling strands of my hair as they listened, a thumb suddenly unplugged to point things out on a page.

As my children grow up, their reading tastes change and these changes are accommodated by their grandmother's generous presents of books, so Anne Fine and Jacqueline Wilson and Michael Morpurgo join the *Gruffalo* and the *Very Hungry Caterpillar* and the *Wild Things* and the *Snowman* so that everybody needs to budge up on the bookshelves to make space and then they need to be piled up, one on top of each other, because all the standing room is taken up. Dust collects between spines so that when I pluck a book to read for the children, I must wipe its cover clean on my jeans.

Books line the walls of my house. They're as important as photographs and pictures in creating a sense of 'home', in telling this family's story, in reminding me of my own history. When we move, my husband bemoans my growing collection. When there is no more space on the shelves, I must pack books in boxes for I cannot bear to part with them. I will keep them, I tell him, 'until the children have homes of their own and then I can parcel up their favourite authors for them to keep', and he rolls his eyes.

When my maternal grandmother Alice died, I inherited over a dozen cartons of her books so that the library I have hung onto from my youth – *Teddy Robinson* and *Anne of*

Green Gables – must make room for the authors my mother read as a child: E. Nesbit and Noel Streatfeild, books whose backs are a little broken and whose pages are floury with age and filled with the scent of other homes and other lives.

'We will not allow your words to be taken from you.' I tell Mum. 'We will teach you to read,' I assure her and she observes me with round eyes full of childlike faith as I promise something I have no idea how to deliver.

*

Research by a team at University College London found that reading the newspaper might reduce the risk of Dementia in women by 34 per cent. The women monitored were from the English Longitudinal Study of Ageing, which includes people born in, or before, the 1950s. The lead author explains that 'at this time, the presence of women in education, and especially in managerial positions, was not very common. So the findings signal that these women are self-teaching and keeping up to date with the world, but do not necessarily have the same education or academic degree.'

'I don't know why my parents never sent me to university. I was clever enough; I should have gone. My life might have been quite different.'

My mother informed herself about the world through words – wherever she found them: in books, a newspaper, magazines.

Sometimes she read to escape the same world.

*

I ask if I can attend the Speech and Language and Occupational Therapy sessions, where Mum learns to navigate her half-blindness, where she will, I assure her, learn to read again. Because I will teach you, I promise, over and over again, 'Just like you taught me,'

'We don't normally allow this,' the family liaison officer informs me stiffly when I ask, 'This' and she waves a hand vaguely as if to prove it hasn't happened before, 'This family-members-sitting-in-on-therapy thing.'

I don't budge.

'She might come back to Africa with me, afterwards, in recovery,' I say, with equal firmness, 'I have to know what I'm doing if I'm going to be able to support her.'

It takes a week. A week of my arriving at the hospital before eight every morning and taking up my position, beside Mum's bed, like a sentry, until after five each evening, a whole week before the occupational therapist gives in: 'Oh well,' she sighs, 'if you're going to sit here all day, you may as well.'

'But,' she warns in a tone that tells me I am testing her, 'only this, not physiotherapy. You cannot attend or observe the physio sessions,' which Mum hates because, she tells me, 'I have to ride a silly bicycle that doesn't go anywhere,' which makes me laugh out loud.

Mum's stroke might not have severed her voice or hamstrung her by deadening movement in her right side or left her choking with dysphagia so she must eat soup and strawberry yogurt under the watchful eye of a spoon-wielding professional. But the damage she did sustain was deep and enduring. And when I can look back, I will know, it was that cruel, fine-tooled extraction that pulled the plug on the precious saved-for-later, it was that which drained her reserve: her lost ability to read.

Because not being able to read a letter or an email means you don't write them. You lose touch with old friends. Not being able to luxuriate in remembering as you read old diary entries means you stop writing a journal and stop flexing your recall. Not being able to read the papers means you lose interest in current affairs. No longer being challenged by a crossword because reading the clues is too hard means you stop testing yourself with *The Times* Cryptic every morning. And not being able to read stories means the place you escaped to for respite is gone.

Having her words stolen from her was like taking the sharpest knife and cutting out the most incisive part of her.

2024

Almost a decade after my mother's stroke, I will stumble upon research that finds a threefold risk of Dementia developing between three and twelve months after stroke. When I contact the author of the study, a stroke neurologist in Canada, he tells me stroke has both immediate and long-term impacts on brain function, and that the elevated risk of Dementia can persist for years.

The presence of risk immediately after stroke wasn't surprising, he said, 'Since there is a direct brain injury which can impact cognition and daily function, and physicians are following up closely with patients in the first year post-stroke, so they're more like to spot signs and make a diagnosis of Dementia.' What was much more surprising, he said, was that the risk persisted during two decades of follow up.

This long-term risk, he explained, 'is probably due to an acceleration of age-related and neurodegenerative pathways. Neuro-inflammation may also play a role.'

I see this now, retrospectively in my mother; her stroke robbed her of her reading – a thief in the night, one day it was there, the next, gone. And that loss eroded those important neural pathways, made them impassable.

'I think,' the Canadian doctor tells me, 'That this could be one of the important ways Dementia risk is elevated after stroke; social activity and intellectual engagement can slow the progression of Dementia. Losing important functions like reading, speaking, or communicating may promote sensory and social isolation and decrease the amount of social and intellectual stimulation. Eventually this may lessen cognitive reserve and make individuals more susceptible to the onset and effects of Dementia.'

It was that cruel, fine-tooled extraction that pulled the plug on the precious saved-for-later, it was that which drained her reserve.

★ ★ ★

The Speech and Language Therapy office is small and airless. There is only space for three chairs and a tiny table. The therapist, Siobhan, sits opposite Mum. I am instructed to take the chair by the door.

The message is unspoken but clear: 'Sit there, sit quietly. Do not interrupt.'

When Mum is settled, Siobhan asks 'Ready?' and holds up a card, with the word 'stove' typed in capitals with an illustration as clue.

Mum, who looks more nervous than ready, considers the card for a moment: 'Oven,' she says.

'No,' says Siobhan kindly, 'Have another go.'

Mum's shoulders slump, just a little, 'Look at the letters,' the therapist encourages, 'one by one.'

Mum sets her jaw, screws up her face in concentration. She can see the card; she just can't make sense of it. She makes several abortive attempts where the s is a c and the v an n. She draws the letters on her palm with a finger as if the feel of them there, on her skin, might draw them out of her head.

Finally she gives up, 'Sorry, I can't get this one.'

When you are told your mother will not be able to read again, because the route between her eyes and her brain is potholed, because the infarct has, explains her neuro, created a roadblock, you imagine there will be some memory of reading to serve as a head start. The alphabet must be in there somewhere, I reason, it just needs to be teased out. It is shocking to discover this is not the case. That every single letter must be relearned. Every F deciphered from a T, each b distinguished from every d.

And Mum's stroke, I realise, has tangled the wiring in her brain; she reads *Cat* quite differently to the way she taught me to read:

Siobhan places a forefinger beneath the word.

Cat.

Mum stares at it, frowns, shifts in her seat. I can't tell if she is shuffling in concentration, because she is uncomfortable. Or because she's getting bored.

Siobhan traces the crescent of the C, 'What's this?' she asks.

'See?' Mum poses, not sounding at all sure. C.

I am puzzled that the letter is not sounded phonetically, as I learned, as I taught my children the alphabet, as Mum taught me:

'Curly Kuh,' they'd have said.

'Why "See" for C?' I wonder.

We struggle through to the 't' which Mum delivers as an 'f'

until the sense of the whole short three-letter word prompts the right ending. C–A–T.

'Cat,' she says, and smiles. A slow, uncertain smile.

'So not Caf then,' and she laughs, 'Silly me!' And I join in, sharing the joke; I want her to know we are in this together.

I can't help myself, 'Siobhan,' (who looks too young to have taught anybody to read) 'can I just ask...?'

Siobhan is not pleased to be Just Asked anything; I have asked quite enough of everybody here already.

I ignore her sit-there-sit-quietly glare, 'Wouldn't it be easier phonetically? I'm just... you know, just saying; wouldn't *buh* for ball be easier than *bee* for ball? That's how I was taught, how I taught my kids, how Mum taught me...' and I trail off then, unsure.

'People don't learn to read like that after a stroke,' Siobhan says shortly, 'They can't.'

But there is another complicating factor that is beginning to show itself: the comprehension of words on a page is handicapped by something else. Mum does not recognise the 'Cat' on Thursday that she managed – eventually – to articulate on Wednesday. It's as if the part of her brain to which new experiences are pasted has been burned, just like the link between her eyes which sees letters and the bit of her brain that recognises them, has been scorched by stroke.

I write this now and I am aghast that I did not consider the part forgetting played in all this then: Mum could not remember the alphabet taught to her as a child. But nor could she remember words taught to her now, this week, in Siobhan's stuffy little office as an adult.

Dementia was whispering.

Perhaps it is – was – as well we suspected nothing – my siblings and I; we refuse to be disheartened – mostly because Mum refuses to be. She bears this extraordinary new determination which we do not recognise, which was never evident in Depression. We are delighted by it and so we hijack every opportunity to exploit it, to encourage Mum to practise her reading. When we walk the hospital grounds with her, which we do every day, we insist she read the signs around those grounds. EXIT. NO ENTRY. PARKING. She cannot see, *seize*, the whole word as we do: as a picture, it must be unpacked into its component parts.

E–X–I–T.

Numbers – oddly – are fine. She remains digit literate; I am astounded one day when I direct her to a small plaque that describes the hospital's history. *1743*, she reads with confidence as she scans the text.

Then, 'What happened in 1743?' And painstakingly, we read about the significance of the date.

Later she asks me, 'Do you think they might have a book about the history of the hospital in the gift shop?'

I promise her I'll have a look.

'Oh good,' she smiles, 'I should like to read all about it.'

And I am so moved by the collision between her old life (when reading was second nature) and her new one (where it cannot be) that I am winded.

Sometimes we try to introduce clever strategies to aid Mum's reading, strategies which do not come from the stiff, young Siobhan, but which my sister, a teacher, introduces me to: visual tricks to help recognise a letter the right way round or the correct way up. Mum's t's are often mistaken for f's, the b's for d's, as if a peculiar sort of dyslexia is manifesting and the alphabet is contorting into confusing shapes.

'See the word, *bed*,' my sister says, and I watch as she writes in her tight hand: 'imagine the b is the sleeper's head and the d the foot of the bed, see how the letters spell, *draw*, the shape – of a bed.' Mum is delighted at the cleverness of this little hand-eye trick.

But when I present the same lesson to my reading student the next day, she falters.

D–E–D, she reads.

The bed is ded.

★

Mum taught us to write too: the tips of our tongues sticking out in concentration, our wrists aching with the unfamiliar effort of holding a pencil as we tried to follow the cursive c's that unfurled like little cresting waves across a page.

And Mum continued to write: even in the years after her stroke, she signed herself with a flourish that rendered her signature both legible and graceful. Mine is neither. The cursive L at the beginning of her first name, the elegant capital S of her second, the letters all evenly delivered.

The last time I watched her do this was as she signed a Power of Attorney. It took six attempts but we got there in the end.

I ask her neurologist (again), 'How come?'

'How come what?' as he seeks clarification for yet another question.

'How come my mum can still write but she can't read?'

'Different connection,' he says, 'one's damaged, one's intact,' and he hurries off before I can begin another interrogation.

Later, I will identify several global experts in Mum's diagnosis: pure alexia – as if we ought to be encouraged by the *pure*, as if it does not spell a blemish, a stain, a bruise, an infarct in her left occipital lobe.

Pure alexia is rare. It is an area of specialist interest because reading is damaged but writing is spared. Central alexia – when both reading and writing are affected – is more common. It seems illogical: that Mum cannot read, cannot even decipher the easy shape of her own name on the page yet she could continue to sign it confidently.

When I don't get what I need from my mother's doctor, I ask Professor Alexander Leff, a neurologist at the National Hospital for Neurology and Neurosurgery in Queen Square, London, and an authority on Mum's diagnosis: 'Why? Why can she write but she can't read?'

He instructs me to close my eyes. I do. He asks me to read a line of text. I can't. Of course, I can't.

He asks me to write my name.

And I can. I do it with ease. Of course I do.

* * *

Mum does not remember to drink. And the instruction to do so which the nurses and I issue daily does not stick, not until thirst sticks Mum's tongue to the roof of her mouth and then it's too late: dehydration causes her blood pressure to plummet which makes her lightheaded and puts her at risk of falls.

Hiss, went Dementia – she does not feel thirst; she cannot remember to drink, are you not listening?

A fresh jug of water is placed by her bedside every morning and refilled throughout the day. But the orderlies who deliver this do not know Mum cannot see it unless it is placed to her left. (The same orderlies who do not know Mum cannot read so leave her a newspaper which she pats and picks up and leafs through and frowns at.)

'Drink Ma,' I urge, moving the jug so she can see it 'You must drink.'

She takes a few sips.

'More,' I insist, then, 'What colour is your pee?' I ask.

'I have no idea,' she says, indignantly, 'I never look at my pee!'

'Well you must start,' I say, 'It needs to be clear,' I explain, 'If it's yellow, it means you're getting dehydrated, you need to drink more.'

We have this conversation every day. Mum forgets her pee must run clear and she forgets to drink. One day, because she has become so dehydrated, her blood pressure falls so low she faints on her way to the loo (to pee her orange pee).

'You must ring your bell if you want to use the bathroom,' the nurses scold her and press the corded bell into her hand, 'Then somebody can help you.' Mum does not remember to do any of it: to ring the bell to go to the loo, to drink, and she cannot read the large red-lettered note I stick with tape and optimism to her table, 'Use your Bell, Drink your Water.'

The nurses tell us again, 'It's not uncommon for short-term memory to be affected for a bit after a stroke.'

Not uncommon. No wonder I wasn't listening.

When she falls a second time, the nurses insist an alarm is fitted to her chair. Each time Mum rises from her seat, a shrill siren screams which makes Mum start. She hates it. But it still does not remind her that she is not meant to leave her seat unaided.

One evening, after I have returned to my temporary home from my hospital vigil, the ward sister phones me, 'Your mum is very distressed, she says she feels like a prisoner, she is insisting we remove the alarm pad from her seat, but we must warn you that if we do this, she could fall and do herself damage, we cannot be liable for that. You must—'

I don't let her finish, 'Take it off,' I say, 'take the alarm off, I'll be responsible.'

The next morning when I walk into her ward, Mum greets me from her chair, naked of its alarm. She has not forgotten she made a scene, 'I think I'm in trouble,' she whispers conspiratorially, 'I made a bit of a fuss last night,' she says with a broad grin.

She may have exposed herself to the risk of falls but she has won a tiny victory in autonomy.

I smile back, 'I heard.'

★

It was only later – much, much later – that I understood what I was noticing then had nothing to do with my mother's stroke and everything to do with the tentacle slide of Dementia.

It seems laughable now: that I could even imagine Mum did not remember the names of all the flowers, could not think what to call her roommates because she had lost her command of the alphabet.

When she asked me over lunch with friends several months after her stroke, 'Where am I again?' I told the astonished audience (*How come she does not know where she is?*) it was because she'd lost her proper nouns along with her reading: 'she's lost everything with a capital letter,' I merrily said, 'The names of all the people and all the places.'

(Isn't it incredible? The things you will make yourself believe? Did I read that somewhere – that the damage wrought of stroke could slice out slender elements of language – proper nouns! – or did I subconsciously invent it, as an excuse?)

But that's not why she didn't know where she was. Of course it wasn't.

She never forgot the name. *Anthea.*

She just forgot it was mine.

* * *

So if my mother's Depression was the culprit for stroke, what place might stroke have had in her subsequent Dementia?

Sometimes I tell myself that if I find the reasons why, I might stand my mother's column of dominoes upright again, order them tidily, which is a fool's game: everybody knows you can't line dominoes up as quickly as you can knock them down.

Strokes happen when the blood supply to an area of the brain is cut off. An infarct, the doctors had said. Infarct from the Latin *infarctus*, from *infarcire* 'to stuff into or with.'

When blood flow is hijacked – because a person has sat too long, say, or because they forgot to drink, and their blood thickens and grows sticky – it can ball as a clot which stuffs itself into an artery like a ping pong ball into a pipe, and blocks it. And when that happens, without a regular, fresh supply of blood, the brain cells around that blockage will be starved of oxygen and they will die.

And messages can't be relayed across dead zones.

* * *

After she has been in rehab for a fortnight, Mum's medical team announce that she is well enough to leave the hospital for a brief outing: 'Just a few hours,' they warn.

My siblings and I plot what we will do with the day. There

is not enough time to leave the city and return without subjecting her to hours in a car, so we opt instead for a Sunday lunch in the nicest restaurant we can afford. We scout those nearby in the week preceding and finally select one after noting it's close enough for Mum to walk to, there are no difficult stairs, it is bright enough that she will see well and we devour reviews to make sure she'll enjoy the food.

But when we get there, I encounter a problem I had not considered: the menu.

How will I manage this with grace?

How will I achieve what I've been trying to do: grant autonomy without accident or embarrassment?

Ought I read her the menu, hand her one to peruse uselessly? The waiter beats me to it, he comes to take our drinks orders and gives us each one of our own to study.

I watch Mum as she opens it. She looks at us closely and tries to navigate to the same page. Afraid I might cry, I say to the table, 'Oh look, that lamb looks delicious – what do you think, Mum?' and, as unobtrusively as I know how, I guide her fingers to the Spring Lamb with Rosemary Roast Potatoes and Pureed Peas.

'Oh yes,' says Mum, 'That *does* sound good.'

When the waiter comes to take our orders, he directs his attention to Mum first, 'Madam?'

I bite my tongue. I do not want to order her lunch for her as I would have done for my children when they were small. Nor do I want her to be embarrassed by giving herself away: that she cannot read.

But Mum has cannily kept her finger beneath her choice and tilts her menu in the direction of the waiter who bends to see what she's pointing at.

'Is that the lamb then, Madam?'

'Yes, yes,' says Mum, 'Lamb, I'll have the lamb,' she nods, 'with the...' her finger hovers and the waiter improvises, 'With the rosemary-roasted potatoes and pureed peas – an excellent choice'

Mum looks up and gives him a broad smile. I can't tell if she's smiling with pride.

Or smiling with relief.

★

I kept questioning my mother's neurologist, when he told me she would not read again, 'But won't the messages learn to get around her brain by a different route, instead of going A B C D E won't they take a detour, and go E B D A C, say?'

He said no. 'No, it doesn't work like that.'

But he was wrong. Mum *did* learn to read again. Not with the same fluency she once read but, many lessons later, some in Siobhan's office, most on my veranda, Mum learned to read at about 30 words a minute. I read at an average 300. Mum probably did too, once. Her brain found its way around the roadblock set up by the clot, and she read. Hesitantly, slowly, but she read. Research suggests this compensatory effect against the pathology of stroke may be because of that precious saved-for-later cognitive reserve.

Years afterwards, a doctor in Australia tells me that while research on cognitive reserve in the context of stroke is not completely understood, preliminary evidence suggests that it has the potential to influence stroke outcomes and recovery. After all, how do you explain how people recover lost ability post-stroke? To talk again, walk, swallow?

Even to read.

So why did my mother's cognitive reserve – which seemed to sustain after stroke for a bit so that she got some reading back – not withstand the pathology of Dementia? If messages managed to circumvent the area of her brain damaged by the necrotising effects of stroke, why did that neural rerouting – that compensation – not grow more robust with practice, not get more efficient, not last?

Because the effect of stroke seeps long after the stroke itself, *due to an acceleration of age-related and neurodegenerative pathways,* partly because, as one doctor explained to me, cerebral blood flow has been interrupted, impeded.

What's good for your heart is good for your head.

Without a circulation, there is no brain function

Add to these physiological insults of stroke my mother's diminished ability to read, a widening separation from the world cleaved by the loss of words, growing isolation, and there was nothing to top that reserve up.

Whether her stroke broke the dam wall of cognitive reserve, or whether Mum's loss of reading hastened its emptying, who knows. But the two together? The two together conspired as a catastrophic brain drain.

2022

My mother used to read Margaret Drabble and Philippa Gregory. Philippa Gregory with her sprawling four-hundred-page historical novels with a vast cast of characters and a stage that spanned centuries; Philippa Gregory who was born in the same city as me, whose father worked for East African Airways as Mum did once – not that any of those connections help us now; Mum can't read about Gregory's *The Other Queen* or *The Last Tudors*. She can't read Drabble and she certainly couldn't read the James Joyce titles she once read – *Ulysses, Dubliners.*

I watch her, puzzling over pages now, squinting, exchanging one pair of spectacles for another, losing patience and asking over and over, 'Where are my reading glasses?'

'Around your neck, Mum.'

'These are not mine,' she shouts, 'I can't read with these.'

How to explain? How to explain when there are so many big words and a lot of confusing language: the right sided hemianopia, the pure alexia. How to explain when a person has no memory of the three months they spent on a rehab ward in a brain injury facility?

How to explain so she does not feel stupid or afraid?

I try to keep it simple: 'You had a stroke, Ma, you mightn't remember, it was a while ago. It means reading is hard.'

Everybody said, 'Get her an iPad'. So we did.

We download the recommended apps. Apps designed to help prop up broken brains. But they are too fast for Mum. Or she can't read the on-screen instructions quickly enough. Or doesn't hear them. Or doesn't understand them.

It becomes an exercise in demoralising frustration.

Then I think: devices are not the answer to everything. I scour my bookshelves. I find one of my eldest daughter's books, *Amelia Jane.* Inside she has written her name and the date: 2000. Amelia Zoe turned seven that year.

I bought it for the title. I bought it for posterity; my own childish bookshelves bore the same story. It was published in 1946. The year my mother turned five. There can be no doubting, given the cover, that this is a children's book. I open it and the text is bold and big and well-spaced.

I press the book into her lap, 'Try this line,' I say:

There was a new toy in the nursery. It was a little telephone. It stood on the nursery bookshelf looking exactly like a real one, but much smaller.

Mum reads so fluently I think she must have guessed at some of the words. But no, I re-read them myself; she has articulated each one precisely as it appears in print. She looks up at me, startled and pleased. 'That was easy,' she smiles.

I don't want her to be offended by the juvenile title, with its puerile illustration on the jacket. So I tell her bluntly: 'Don't think I am patronising you, Mum: it's not *what* you read, it's *how* you read. And if we can build up your speed, you'll get better: practice makes perfect.'

(It doesn't by the way – we tried, we practised every day, the same passages, over and over and over until my eyes began to droop with the boredom of it all. I sometimes wondered why Mum didn't get bored too – now I know why.)

Two hours later, two hours of silence, no exasperated tapping of a screen, no cross 'Oh shucks' and deep sighs, no shouting about the wrong glasses, and she has 'read' 158 pages.

I know she cheated. She has not read all of those pages. She has slipped her bookmark further into the book – by accident or design, does it matter? No, I tell myself, it does not. What matters is her immersion in the trying.

But reading is more complicated than words on a page, it is about context and comprehension and who's who and holding the narrative in your head. Mum cannot do that for she cannot tell me about the story she has just read.

Still, I notice she begins to take *Amelia Jane* with her everywhere, to and from her room, as if carting some security blanket with her, some shred of her former unbroken self.

* * *

When I think of my mother, I think of her in four parts – a quartet, scored, scarred by illness and injury so that separate elements of her are revealed one by one. Separate, unexpected elements at separate unexpected times of her, *my*, life.

Sometimes I think of Mum as an exhibit of abstract art where pieces of her are where they shouldn't be – lips in the middle of her face, say, or a multi coloured portrait, a Picasso, whose features are exaggerated: one enormous eye in the centre of her forehead or mismatching ears. Sometimes I think she presents as a collage where words and pictures jumble to try to form the whole, a whole that can be difficult to navigate, 'What is that, *exactly*?' you ask yourself as you study it, craning your neck and squinting as you try to fathom the message.

Which way is up, which way down?

And as the moving parts of my mother's mind shaped her differently, so she had to learn to pick her way around this new person that evolved, had to learn to accommodate a life that looked, felt, quite different. And we, we who love her and live with her and know her – or at least knew the most recent manifestation of our mother that presented – we must learn to understand her all over again; we have to reconstruct our connection with her as she rebuilds herself.

We have to find our way back to her.

My well mother anchored us. She was the slight but solid centre of our lives, a compass so we knew which way we were headed. She was the fulcrum of a circle: she kept things going round, on an even keel.

In Depression and Stroke, my mother was still there, misshapen, but reachable. She still knew who we were – who I was – and who we were to her. When she stopped knowing, and even though I swam as hard as I could, she drifted out of reach. And it felt then as if a tide had risen and was lifting her off.

Chapter 9: A Rising Tide

Ireland, July 2021

I almost can't bear to ask my brother: 'Does she know I'm coming? Does she know it's me?'

'I think so,' he says in his measured, kind, careful way, afraid to cause hurt or elevate expectations.

We are driving home to his from Dublin, summer green slips past. The roads are quiet. Ireland is still under house arrest. Freedom Day isn't for another week and a half. Long enough for me to sit out my mandatory Covid incarceration before I scoop Mum up and take her to my sister's in England for a month. Long enough, I hope, for her to know me again; it is eighteen months since she saw me to forget who I was. How will she remember me now?

'She a bit nervous,' my brother says, 'She's been flicking through old calendars,' he adds.

In recent years, every Christmas, my sister and her children created bespoke calendars for Mum, illustrated with images of family members – children, grandchildren, siblings, parents – 'I think she's familiarising herself with who's who.'

I see Mum before she opens the door, her shape is puddled behind an opaque glass pane, she comes towards me like a swimmer rising from under water.

And then the door opens and she is there. It takes her a

moment, an instant where she looks distant and confused and then something like recognition floods her face.

I speak before she does. Just in case she needs reminding, 'Hello Mum! How lovely to see you!'

And I envelop her small frame in a hug. She is stooped – more stooped than I remember – and tiny and she feels brittle beneath my embrace.

I cannot decide later if I use this word – brittle – because I notice a stiffening of her back as I put my arms around her. Or whether I chose the word because I felt as if she might crack if I hugged too tight.

'Hello Anthea,' she smiles.

★

In the camera-off Skype calls that I have had with Mum while we've been Coronavirus-cleaved apart, I have told her about the summer holiday plans I am making.

'I'm booking a house, Mum,' I say, 'We'll all congregate there.'

'Oh, how lovely,' says Mum, 'I shall look forward to that.'

She does not ask who the 'all' are.

I tell Mum the same thing every time I call.

And her response is unchanging, always: fresh delight, as if she has never heard this plan before. Her enthusiasm never dims.

I tell her where we are planning to go. 'The south coast of England,' I say.

I tell her who is going to join us. Her children – and I speak their names. I include myself: 'Me, Anthea.' Our children, 'All your grandchildren,' I say (I don't bother with names – there are too many for that). 'Your sister,' I say, whose name Mum never forgets. Ever.

My brother, before I arrive and when I share these grand holiday plans with him over the phone, assures me Mum is still mobile.

'Except I'm not sure how well she'd cope with stairs,' he warns, when I describe the Airbnb I have my eye on, 'Probably not a whole flight,' he warns. (He lives with Mum in a safely single-storey bungalow.)

'How steep are they, the stairs?' My brother asks now.

I contact the Airbnb host: 'Sorry, another question. How steep are the stairs?'

'Not especially,' she responds, 'but they are quite narrow.'

'And make sure there's a handrail,' adds my brother as an afterthought.

'Is there a handrail?' I ask the host in a third – or is it a fourth? – email. I can tell, from her increasingly curt responses, that she is getting fed up.

She messages back: a one-word response: 'No.'

I strike the house from my list.

Beach houses are at a premium this summer. Everybody is staycationing in case the government forces another lockdown. Except me. I'm not staycationing. I'm travelling halfway around the world to make sure this holiday happens. Jumping through quarantine hoops as I go. Africa to lenient eastern Europe to less lenient Ireland to England, decontaminating as I go, ten days here, ten days there.

'I'll spend some time with you first, if that's okay,' I say to my brother.

'Sure,' he says; he knows why I need to do this.

I tell Mum, 'I'll have a few days with Rob and family first, you know, just to catch up… and then you and I can head off.'

'Oh how lovely,' says Mum again.

She doesn't know why. And she doesn't know I'm lying.

I do that a lot now. Lie.

Spending time with my brother when I pick Mum up is so that she can acclimatise to me.

What if I get there and she refuses – again – to believe I am her daughter, refuses to come away with me? Imagines she's being abducted by a stranger?

I ask the agent at the cottage rental business, 'What happens if I have to cancel?'

I tell him I am anxious that Covid may present obstacles which might mean we cannot take our reservation up: 'What if somebody tests positive?' I ask.

He says there is provision for such an event.

What would he say if I told him that the reason I might have to cancel is because one of our party refuses to come away with me because she has forgotten I am her daughter? Again.

I add a note to my list: 'Check travel insurance for cancellation policies.'

My brother pings me a message: 'Mum has developed a tendency to wander at night.'

At night, when the layout of an alien house will be dangerous for Mum even if the stairs are wide with a gentle gradient and bound by a handrail. What if she takes a tumble in the dark, I worry, on a nocturnal mission for tea or to the loo or because she thinks she is on a ship and tries to get off?

I strike every double story cottage from my search.

I Google 'bungalows by the sea.' I find one.

It has two king size beds.

'Could we replace one of the kings with twins?' I ask the host. But I have already asked him about how close the cottage is to the beach. I have scrutinised the photos of the bathroom and asked about shower access. Mum cannot step into a bath to shower. I am not sure she could heave herself up out of a tub. Her ablution requirements are specific. I want the host to understand this without spelling out how damaged she is. I do not want him to turn us down because he thinks my mother is an almost incontinent geriatric. Even if she is. I have asked about his cancellation policy, the view and whether there are any steps at all in the property.

'No,' he says.

'No view or no steps?' I seek to clarify,

He doesn't write back; he is tired of me with my window shopping. He imagines he knows why I'm being difficult. He'd never guess.

And then it dawns on me. Mum will remember nothing of her holiday within days of returning home. She will remember only the hour she is in – her present is what counts, her past will go the way of all memories; her days will dissolve to nothingness.

And suddenly I know, this holiday is for us, for me: this holiday is the last I'll have with a mother who might know something of her history so that occasionally she will bob hopefully back into sight.

My – our – memories of it are what count.

I scrap the idea of beachside Airbnbs with a view. Instead, we all go to my sister's small house in a tiny Wiltshire town where the local supermarkets and short walks are familiar, where my sister and I can sleep safely close to Mum, ears cocked for the slightest sound of night-time wandering, where we can barricade stairs

It is perfect.

*

Briefly then, that summer, in Ireland, before I whisk Mum away on Freedom Day when Shannon Airport is full of press taking pictures of people making a break for it, Mum and I become shyly reacquainted.

Every day we walk. Sometimes she walks confidently: 'Yes, that's right, it's this way now,' she says, pointing out our direction as she navigates familiar paths, recognises landmarks, orients herself again and again in a place she's lived for years. She guides me with something like pride. She may not always know who I am, but she knows I'm a visitor here. That I need showing the ropes. I find her polite solicitude poignant.

One afternoon we walk through a patch of forest which is strung with wildflowers. I had not noticed them when I walked the path alone first and fast to recce it for obstacles and trip hazards before I walk the same route with Mum later, pretending it's the first time I've ever walked it: 'No, I've never been this way before, Mum, you show me.' I don't notice the flowers until I walk the same walk with Mum and she points them out.

She stops and traces blossom that drips from a bush with her fingertips. The blooms are bridal white as they erupt from foliage that flushes new green. I watch Mum's face as she picks one and puts it to her nose to inhale its scent.

Then: 'Look,' she says, 'These leaves haven't turned pink yet; they will.'

And I remember her passion for garden centres and how I could ask, 'What's this called, Mum?'

And she always knew.

* * *

There is an analogy in Dementia that speaks of bookcases. If books are memories, the oldest are on the bottom shelf, the newer ones at the top. If the bookcase were shaken, or moved from one side of a room to another, the volumes on the top shelf would tip to the floor. The top shelf books represent a sufferer's short-term memory, the ones solidly at the bottom are the oldest, and their most secure recollections.

My mother's parents – and the sister she has been close to all her life whose name she never forgets – those are Mum's bottom-shelf books. They stay put.

It's the top-shelf ones that can be problematic; when they tip to the floor, it's hard to put them back. You mightn't be able to reach that high – I have shelves that regularly call for a chair in order that I might examine what's up there (amongst the dust and dead flies). Or you mightn't be able to find a book's rightful place. The metaphorical books which are too difficult to put back are the memories that cannot be reinstated. Me, my brother and sister, definitely all our children, we have all tipped from the top shelf. Mum has no idea now where we fit. She can't slot us back into place.

All that anchors Mum is the weight of the bottom-shelf books. That's where Bombay sits, its spine cracked and dusty. Where her parents are. Her younger-by-18-months sister. Where we sometimes find a memory of plants and flowers rooted.

I will puzzle often: if I grew from a seed inside her, why does she not know the adult I have grown into?

'Because,' a doctor explains, 'she does not expect to see an older face on the daughter she birthed; she cannot compute this fact of growing up, growing old.'

Am I there then as a child, where she imagines I belong, still sturdily held in those low shelves as a little girl, plump-bodied, hair the colour of straw, small freckled face round and raised up to my mother?

Is that what she expects to see? Not the lined one looking down at her as she leans against me for support when she bends to inspect a flower.

I ask Mum one day, 'Is it frightening, Mum, the no-memory thing? Or confusing?'

I ask because she remarks upon her memory often: 'My memory these days,' as she slaps her forehead in frustration when a name eludes her.

She considers my question for a moment.

'No,' she says, 'It is neither of those things. But it means I have to be completely sure about something. In case I get it wrong, you see.'

And I think, 'There! There it is,' in that instant, I have understood the loss of confidence in loading dishwashers and putting away clean glasses. She can't remember what some things do or where they go; she does not want to get it wrong.

We are almost home when I see apprehension cloud her face. She is lost. She stops, her head turning this way and that, the little posy of flowers she has collected as we walked drooping despondently in her hand.

She does not imagine that I know my way: I don't live here, after all. She will not ask me, I am her guest.

And I don't want to prompt her. I want her to recognise the landmarks, the same ones we have already passed today. The same landmarks she has passed countless times in the years she has been here. I want to know that even if she cannot place me or my dead dad, she can still place herself.

'Let's keep walking, Mum,' and I nudge her over the road so that we are pointed in the right direction.

Suddenly, then, she knows where she is; I see recognition and, given her lack of faith in my navigation as a newbie to these parts, relief, 'Oh, look! We're home,' she smiles.

★ ★ ★

Mum's hair is long and white and yellowed with age at the ends. She ties it up in a ponytail. She hasn't washed it for weeks. (I don't know yet that she can't anymore). And she hasn't been to a hairdresser since before the first lockdown.

'It feels wet,' she says.

It needs a good wash. I laugh, 'Let me help.'

I watch her later, as she combs it out.

'Shall we get it cut?' I suggest. 'It's very long.'

'Yes,' she says, 'Yes, let's.'

★

The morning of her hair appointment, I find her in front of a mirror, her fingers spread beneath her eyes; 'I look terrible, I am so ugly,' she wails, 'I have holes in my face' and she points to them: the hollows below her cheek bones.

I tell her, 'Once all that long hair is gone, your face will look plumper.'

She is intrigued by this idea, she wants to understand why: why will she look less thin with shorter hair?

And as I try to explain the new perspective of shorter cuts on the shape of a face, I am struck by her vanity; I find it a hopeful thing.

In the dictionary, the word – *vanity* – describes something empty, of no value and yet here, here on my vanishing mother it speaks to something precious: she still minds the way she looks. And somehow the desire to preserve the way she used to look speaks to saving the person she used to be.

And I am touched by her trust that I can weave the magic I have made her believe I can, that with a haircut I will transform her into someone younger and fill up the holes in her face. If only it were so easy to fill up the holes in her memory. If only I could do that.

Caped up, she sits at the hairdresser's station. I see her worried eyes wide above her mandatory mask.

I don't know if she's anxious because she's in a strange place – brought here by a sometimes-strange woman. Or because she isn't sure what she ought to do – should she be doing something? Saying something? Asking for something? Should she just keep sitting here and wait?

I have filled my phone with old photographs of a younger mother, one with all her memories intact wearing a chic gamine cut and broad smile. She considers the images on the screen that I tip in her direction.

'Gosh,' she says, 'look at me!'

'This short, Mum? Do you want it cut like this?'

'Yes,' she is certain.

I show the hairdresser, I hold out my phone, 'Like this,' I say.

'Really?' she asks, 'That short?' And she holds Mum's hair up from the nape of her neck, 'All this will go, are you sure?'

Perhaps she imagines this daughter – who manhandles her mother with her blind side and her disappearing past into the chair, steering her round trip hazards – is more managing than minding.

Mum is certain, 'Yes,' she nods, 'yes.'

And so the hairdresser begins to cut and great handfuls of hair fall to the floor and gather at her feet and look like ash against the soot-black of the tiles.

I watch and I laugh, 'You'll feel quite lightheaded after this, Mum' and I feel a weight dissolve from my shoulders. The last time I took Mum to the hairdresser was before the

Christmas she forgot who I was. She was full of fury and railed at my trying to deceive her into the stylist's chair. In the end we only managed a wash that day. But today she is full of anticipation at a new look, soothed by the touch of hands upon her head, as the young girl who shampoos her hair does it with such sweet attentiveness, and the hairdresser primps and snips and tilts Mum's head forward so that she can cut close to her skin, behind her ears.

And I watch the shape of my mother's brilliant head re-emerge, the soft, elegant, perfect curve of her skull, her neck lengthens and her gauntness is gone, her face newly rounded.

Compliments abound when she is done. The girls in the salon gather round, 'You look fabulous,' they say and Mum beams and pats her hair and steals surreptitious glances at herself in the mirror and graciously accepts compliments, 'Thank you, thank you so much. It's lovely.'

I leave a tip so large, I notice the hairdresser's eyes well.

We walk home and I swear Mum seems taller, walks with a brisker step. Holds her head a little higher. And all afternoon she keeps smiling at her reflection every time it catches her and smiles back. She has blossomed into somebody she was years ago. After supper that night, Mum sits around the table until eleven, savouring a glass of wine, listening to the stories of my young niece and nephew, not always following their fast, contemporary chat but listening with such interest, her curiosity alight; I can see it burn from her eyes.

And then she offers a story of her own, about her brother, one I have heard before. She tells it again now and it is pitch perfect, delivered with detail and colour and expression as she gestures and laughs and entertains in a way she once did easily.

And I know: she is in there, Mum is still in there. All it took was a haircut. Today, that's all it took.

★

I worried about the flight, that 19 July flight to freedom. I worried Mum would balk at the eleventh hour. That she would refuse to travel with me. That our arrival the other side may be too bewildering.

And the morning we are due to make the short trip over the sea from the west coast of Ireland to London, some of my worries threaten to manifest. Mum complains of nausea and keeps sinking back into her bed when I try to urge her up, 'Get up, Ma, get up, or we'll miss our plane.'

This is how anxiety has always shown itself in Mum: something tangible to pin the intangible upon. 'I feel sick' means, 'I feel worried.' I can translate Depression-speak. I must learn the language of Dementia now.

I peel her nightdress off, coax her into trousers, a blouse, ease her feet into shoes and tie her laces. I reassure her that I have packed everything she needs, as I have reassured her several times a day in the week before this big adventure. My brother drives us the short distance to the airport and dispatches us with his usual calm and kindness. I see a shadow cross Mum's face, 'When will I see you again?'

'I will come and fetch you,' he promises. He is her cornerstone for now. I am beginning to understand what courage it must take to leave this rock of familiarity, to loosen her grip on the handle of the known and step into what must be a void. It is such a leap of faith. She has not left the house for more than a brief walk, the odd doctor's appointment, in almost 18 months. Now she accepts my hand – the hand of a sometimes stranger – as I walk her onto the escalator so that my brother shrinks and then disappears beneath her as she waves, like a child.

But her nerves leave her then and she is full of questions, a commentary that runs on a loop, 'When will our plane leave? Do you think all these people are on our train? I wonder where they are all going? Are you sure we're in the right place? When will our plane leave...? How long will we be on the train?' My well mother's default was always one of curiosity, her best advice: 'Ask questions.' Her face now is animated by wanting to know. She cannot, will not, remember, but she wants to know *now.*

She is thrilled to board the plane, smiles at every other passenger as we make our way down the aisle. I fasten her seat belt. She examines the laminated safety instructions then tucks them back into the pocket of the seat in front of her when she realises she can't make head or tail of them. Instead she turns to look out of the window. Above her mask her eyes are bright and smiling; I see excitement reflected there. She delights in take-off. She points out the shrinking fields, toy-town houses, the Irish Sea which on this summer's day is ironed smooth by steam-hot heat. She exclaims at the bump back to earth as we land and laughs out loud. She insists on walking, declines a wheelchair, even as we trail our way through the bowels of Gatwick Airport dragging suitcases. She is so eager, so trusting as she walks with me. I had not expected this. I had expected resistance. Even refusal. Definitely a dragging of feet. But she rises to this challenge with energy and grace.

'Thank you,' she says as the taxi driver relieves her of her bag, and 'Thank you so much,' when he opens her door and she slides gratefully into the rear seat and sinks into it.

She rises to all this with courage. It must be like being led blindfold. She has no idea where she is going, or – especially – who she is going there with.

Do you know what that might feel like? I don't.

But I imagine it might be like stepping off a cliff.

Wiltshire, July 2021

My sister's new home is Mum-friendly and bright. There is a kitchen large enough that she can sit in there, on the comfortable chair my sister has bought for the purpose, and watch us as we cook or wash up or listen to our chat. She is content to do that, to try to work out, from what we say, who we are and how we are all connected. Sometimes she asks, 'Are you my eldest daughter?' And I laugh, and say, 'And your favourite one,' as my sister gives me a shove, 'Hey!'

'It's easier with two of us, isn't it?' my sister confides on a walk.

It is. But not for the reasons you might imagine; this is not about the physical heft of Mum, not yet, or even shared responsibility when patience is worn. It is easier to carry the weight of Mum's forgetting with another because it's easier to carry on a conversation.

Dementia is eroding my mother's ability to be the excellent company she once was. She has little history to share now, few stories to recount, whatever I tell her will not stick, so our conversations are circuitous, our dialogue hiccups with confusion. There are pregnant pauses filled with the weight of wondering what I can say next, pauses which are always aborted by my mother's forgetting. If you listened in to a two's-company conversation you'd quickly understand something was wrong from my mother's repetition or non-responses.

As a little crowd of three we work, as three my mother need only be an appreciative audience to mine and my sister's banter. We can include her peripherally – 'Isn't that right, Mum?' or

'What a cheeky mare she is, Mum,' or 'Listen to how bossy my sister is,' and Mum has only to chuckle or acquiesce or argue with the shake of her head. If you eavesdropped on this conversation, you'd never know anything was wrong. If you were just two with Mum, the gaps and holes would reveal themselves; with three it's easier to patch them up as we go along. With three we can almost pretend everything's normal.

I soon find in this distillation of time, this single precious month, that everything is intensified by a peculiar piquancy, the ordinary elevated to extraordinary. I can't be sure if this is because we understand we must make every single second of it count, or because our lives feel arrested with Mum's memory, but there is something heady about that summer.

Every morning when we wake, my sister and I make tea in the kitchen, we gather up our mugs, and one for Mum with a tin of biscuits and climb back up the short staircase that we instruct Mum every day never to attempt on her own. We clamber into her big bed then, the double bed my sister has surrendered for now – all three of us. We gather like schoolgirls, laughing and teasing and storytelling. Mum's face is radiant with delight and something like disbelief, as if she has been included in a party she never imagined she'd be invited to (for who are these people to ask her?). I sit beside her and admire her nightdress. She smooths a sleeve as she considers the pattern and the softness of the cotton.

'Anthea gave it to me.'

I smile, 'What excellent taste Anthea has.'

And my sister rolls her eyes.

I find emotions are more potent – as if every single one is stretched clingfilm-thin. So either I laugh until I weep or I tip close to sadness and want to cry.

Sometimes I find the close-to-surface hilarity startling.

Mum rises from the sofa for bed one evening and complains her knee is stiff and sore. I tell her what I tell her every time she rises from a chair with the same complaint: 'Move it Ma, move it, swing it back and forth,' and she does then, and it loosens.

But this night I am seized by the ridiculous, I clutch her hand and say, 'Here Ma. Watch me, like me,' and I begin to sing as I swing my leg, 'Put your left leg in, your left leg out,' as I bend it from the knee, 'In out, in out, shake it all about' and Mum tries to keep up and we both laugh so hard that I am bent double. When we walk then, joints loosened, towards the staircase up to bed, I prompt Mum to grab the handrail with both hands except, slip of the tongue, I tell her to grab the stairs instead.

Mum drops to her knees and makes to crawl up the stairs. For a moment, I am appalled, 'What's she doing?' It is only when I correct myself, 'Not like that,' I say, 'I meant the rail,' that I realise she is convulsed with laughter.

She is playing with me.

She is still there, she is still sometimes, somewhere, in there. And when I see her, it is as if the dust and cobwebs that Dementia is stringing across her brain are blown briefly away. As if something has pierced through the hardness of all this and excavated some old part of her. And it is like finding a diamond in the rough when that happens. There she is: there's my sparkling, brilliant, mother.

We tease her often, my sister and I. On a walk, we urge, 'Faster Mum, faster,' or 'Shall we swing you between us like you and Dad used to?' and I threaten, as I raise her arm: 'Like this, wheeeeeee'!

'Don't you dare,' she laughs.

Sometimes we make as if to push her up hills by planting our flattened palms against her lower back and she laughingly protests. Or we tell her we are walking five miles this afternoon and she grinds to a halt, stops dead in her tracks and announces, 'Then I shall turn back right now and walk home on my own,' so that we collapse, giggling, 'Ma, you'll never find the house!'

She wouldn't. She often can't find the bathroom. Or the kitchen. Or the front door.

Once I said, 'Sorry Mum, I shouldn't laugh.'

'Why not?' she said, 'If you can't laugh, what is there?'

★

I begin to think, that summer, of my mother's fragmenting memory as a jigsaw puzzle. One that has been broken into a thousand tiny pieces. Nothing makes sense anymore. Once upon a time, the picture was whole and clear, sharp-edged with all the corners in place, and then it was knocked. Dozens of pieces fell to the floor, were kicked beneath the sofa. Nobody will find them now. Certainly not Mum, even when she tries really hard, she can't reach them. I think my father's face is there, hidden from view. Sometimes the shape of the rest of us doesn't fit into the shape Mum expects it to. She moves the pieces about, sifts through them, trying to find what she's looking for. And sometimes she does.

But mostly she doesn't.

★

We have unearthed a pack of playing cards, a regular deck but the back of each bears the photograph of a family member. (Like the calendars, something everyday-ordinary that we hoped would orient Mum in the who's-who of her family).

I can tell they have never been used. They don't have the necessary softness to yield to a good shuffle. Their backs crack when I try.

Mum watches me as I line them up on a table for a game of Patience.

'What silly cards,' she says, 'I've never seen cards like that, with people on them,' she scoffs.

I ignore her comment and keep counting cards.

Then I say, 'Do you know how to play Patience, Ma?'

'Nope,' she says shortly.

I pretend not to notice when she starts to watch me as I match numbers and suits on my 'silly' cards. And I watch Mum's body tip forward, lean in. Tentatively, she begins to join in.

'Could you put that one there?'

'Oh well done, Ma, I hadn't seen that; thank you.'

And then she says, sounding surprised, 'I recognise some of these faces!'

So I prompt: 'Who am I with here?'

'That's my Mum!' she says, delighted to spot somebody she knows (the subtext of her tone: *what a surprise to find my* ***mother*** *amongst these strangers*).

'Yup, that's right, that's Gran – your mum. And these are my daughters – your granddaughters.'

'You taught me all the card games I know, Gran,' says my grown-up son who is watching. Mum looks thrilled: that she, who feels so frail and lost now, could have taught this strapping young man anything.

'Did I really? Well, that's rather wonderful isn't it?'

'Indeed,' my kind son smiles, 'It *is* rather wonderful.'

My daughters travel with a deck of cards everywhere they go. I have often watched them on the floor of an airport terminal, studying a fan of cards in their hands with careful intent. Mum taught them to play too: Go Fish, Rummy, Sevens. And in those lessons she gifted them an old-fashioned occupation; they're never bored with a pack of cards which they shuffle like pros.

'Shall we play another?' I suggest, as I scoop the cards up.

'Oh yes,' says Mum, 'let's!'

'We'll play until we've outwitted the deck,' I say. So we do – best of five; we win.

A game of Patience morphs into one of Memory – Mum needs more of one, I need more of the other.

★

If I imagined that summer would gift us something important to remember, I was right. But it does something else: it focuses a lens on everything Mum is losing – has already lost. And it's not just her memory. We are acclimatising to her increasing incontinence.

My sister and I begin to find damp knickers stuffed under the bed or at the back of drawers. Mum only understands what has happened too late, there is still enough of her to feel embarrassed by these 'accidents' so she hides the evidence. This is worse, we agree, than if she did not register at all. We whip soiled underwear into the washing machine before Mum stumbles upon it looking for a clean pair, for between one accident and the next, she forgets. It is one of a tiny handful of meagre and minuscule (for they are small and few) mercies of this horrid illness, that sometimes the forgetting spares a person humiliation.

Sometimes Mum expresses distress or frustration at not making it to the loo on time. I tell her it's normal for women her age, especially for women who've had children, I say (even if you aren't sure who – or where – those children are, they've still ripped through you). I learn that if not making it to the bathroom on time starts with a failing ability to locate the bathroom as internal maps are frayed as spatial awareness goes, it gets worse when galloping cognitive decline means the messaging system between brain and bladder and then brain and bowel starts to break down.

In the end, months after that summer, living with me by then, I will lower Mum to the loo and she will look at the contents of her diaper and appear startled: 'Oh look,' she will say in astonishment. Subtext, 'I wonder where *that* came from.' And there is no shame and there it is again: that tiny merciful hand of this cruel disease.

We make nothing of this new development except to understand we need to accommodate a physiological challenge. The next time we go to the supermarket, my sister navigates our shopping trolley towards the sanitary products aisle. We pick up three packets of incontinence pads as nonchalantly as we can and place them in the bottom of our cart. It feels much bigger than it looks. If you saw us, you'd never imagine that this was two girls accepting their mother is getting sicker. We are quiet for a bit after that. Our usual banter abandons us.

We add a six pack of Guinness for Mum and a bag of the blandest crisps to eat with them so as not to irritate the sensitive lining of her mouth, and we head home.

★

One evening towards the end of those halcyon days of that summer, I leave Mum to take a shower.

'Do you know how to use it?' I ask her.

'Of course I do,' she says.

'Well I'm just here, outside, reading. If you need me, call me.'

'I will,' she promises.

Twenty minutes later and concerned, I crack the bathroom door open. The steam I expected from a hot shower is not in evidence and Mum is dressed.

'Did you have a nice shower, was it warm enough?'

'Oh no, I didn't have a shower. I decided I didn't really need one'

'I think a shower would be a good idea, Mum,' I press.

'Well, I don't know how to use the taps, they aren't like the ones I'm used to.'

'I told you to call me, Ma, I could have put it on for you, adjusted the temperature until it was just right.'

'How could I? You were out on a walk.'

'No I wasn't, I was right here.'

She sighs as if in defeat, then: 'Who are you, anyway?'

And there it is: another jarring too-steep step down.

I tell my sister when I do go out on a walk, 'This will be our last, I think, our last summer of Mum.'

It is.

But we will tell ourselves often afterwards: at least we had *that* summer. One precious month, which Mum captures every essence of in the few words she writes in my sister's Visitor's Book when she returns to Ireland with our brother. She uses the word 'enjoyable' four times to describe her stay. Enjoyable and 'interesting' because she met lots of new relations.

She signs off with, 'Lots of love from your Aunt Lala.'

And two years later, my brother will stand up in a church and he will call that summer 'Mum's Last Hurrah.'

★ ★ ★

There must come a time when every family affected by Dementia has to have The Conversation. The Conversation about what to do with Mum. Or Dad. The Conversation that must be had now because you didn't have it then, when you should have done: Back when the parent in question was still able to articulate a choice, when they still had opinions about things that mattered. Still bore agency and autonomy.

And though my siblings and I did not have that conversation *with* our mother, it was Mum who unwittingly steered us towards a decision.

Years earlier, long before Dementia was a part of any conversation, long before the word was even a part of our vocabulary, when Mum was whole and in command of all her faculties: on top of her correspondence, in control of her finances and her bladder. When she knew her children. Back then, Mum used to visit an elderly friend in a nursing home. Sometimes I would accompany her.

The nursing home, in an old vicarage, was set in pretty grounds in a quaint village. You entered through a heavy green door; I had to lean my shoulder into it to open it. Then I stood aside and held the door open for Mum before settling into the safety of her slipstream to follow her. She came here often; she bore a confidence that I did not. The vacant expressions of some residents frightened me as they stared from where they sat in ranks of wheelchairs pushed up against a wall as if to watch television but not seeing anything. The air was heavy with the smell of whatever was for lunch, talcum powder and disinfectant. I didn't know better yet; I wrinkled my nose behind Mum.

It was clear, the moment Mum entered her friend's room,

that she brought something like sunshine. Her elderly friend – whose cognition was still sound but who suffered mobility issues – responded to Mum's arrival with evident delight. Her face split by the broadest smile, she reached up to grasp Mum's hand and turned her cheek to receive Mum's kiss upon skin which I knew, for I had pressed my lips to it too, had the peculiar floury softness of an elderly person's complexion. Mum fussed over her, making tea and opening biscuits and the old lady kept up a stream of chat. Mum responded to everything she said as if it were the most interesting thing she'd heard all week.

I watched and I thought to myself, this single hour out of my mother's day is what helps make this old lady's week – an hour's injection as prophylaxis against boredom or loneliness or fears of being abandoned for the next seven days. Basking in the glow of Mum's attention, I saw the old lady blossom in that short hour, her skin pinked with the exhilaration of it all.

When it was time to go, Mum rinsed the mugs we'd used, plumped the cushions we'd leant against, gathered up her bags, kissed the old lady goodbye and promised to be back soon. And we left, back down the stairs to the high care floor below where the television was still shouting at its silent and apparently uncomprehending viewers, and back outside through the big green door.

I always felt relieved to get out into the fresh air.

On one occasion when we left, as the heavy door slammed shut behind us, Mum said, 'Please God, never let me be in a place like this.'

Please God, never let me be in a place like this.

I heard *place like this;* I understood she meant, 'Never put me into nursing care, look after me in my own – or your – home.'

It didn't occur to me until years later that she might have meant she'd rather be dead than *like this.*

Please God, never let me **be** *like this.*

★

Ant and I have had The Conversation.

He used to say, before we understood anything about Dementia, 'If I ever lose my marbles, just hit me over the head.'

Which is crazy. Because I can't. And I couldn't. It would be unlawful. And it would be unthinkable.

His approach is more thoughtful now; the experience of living with somebody who has Alzheimer's forces you to rethink opinions long-held.

And to think again – with careful deliberation – about possible future scenarios. Mostly because it makes them real, drags them into sharper focus.

'If you could just end your life, if you had Dementia, if – when – you felt your quality of life wasn't worth it…' he says.

'But you can't,' I remind him, 'By the time it's not worth living, you won't know it's not worth living. You'll have lost everything – not just your memories, but maybe your ability to walk, shower, use the loo, feed yourself, understand anything, say a word. You definitely won't be able to tell if life is worth living.'

I think of Amy Bloom's husband, Brian Ameche. She describes an agonising choice in her memoir. Ameche – diagnosed with early onset Dementia – opted to end his life at Dignitas even though it was still mostly a life worth living most of the time. But the choice had to be made while he still had the agency to make it himself.

And I think of Julianne Moore's confusion in *Still Alice* when she is unable to follow the suicide instructions she left for herself long before early onset Alzheimer's undid her.

By the time you've lost that quality of life – your memories, stories, balance, the comprehension to understand something on the television, follow a conversation, by the time you're incontinent, cannot feed yourself the food you can no longer taste – you'll also have lost your powers of reasoning. You will have lost executive function, and you'll have lost the ability to follow anything like Moore's carefully scribed and filed directions.

You'll probably also have lost the wish to die. In Dementia, I was occasionally startled by my mother's vice-like grip on life. As if in losing higher cognition, her primal instinct to survive hadn't just remained, it had mushroomed, grown urgent in the absence of everything else. She grew to fret about the tiniest ailment. When paranoia became a feature of her days, she became frightened people were trying to poison her. Including me.

'If you kill me,' she wailed one day, 'I will come right back and kill you.'

These were not the words of a woman who wanted to end her life.

So if you cannot execute the necessary to end it yourself and, given it's illegal for anybody else to do it for you, what to do?

My husband and I ponder this quandary for a while.

Then I say, 'I don't want you to look after me.'

I mean, I don't want *him* to be the one bathing me, feeding me, dressing me, wiping me…

I don't want the man I have lived with for decades – my husband, companion, partner, lover, friend – at the raw end of this. I want his memories of us unsullied by a disease that starts with forgetting. My mother's Dementia has worn her away so that there's almost nothing left, and at the same time, it has eroded my memories of her. 'Death by a thousand cuts,' my husband calls it.

'A care home or a paid carer,' I say, 'if we – you – can afford it. Just not you.'

He agrees, 'Me too,' he says, 'not you.'

'I don't want our children looking after me either,' I say.

'Me neither,' he nods.

'Make sure,' I urge my husband, 'I have a cat to sit on my lap, a view to gaze at, a dog at my feet, a glass of wine, or two, in the evening and roll me the odd cigarette.' And I can taste the liquorice paper we used to roll our tobacco with back then. Back then when we were young and immortal and reckless.

'Make sure I have a prescription that manages my mood. Don't let me be sad. Don't let me be scared. If I can't sleep at night, make sure I can.'

'Take me off all my other prescription meds,' my husband says: 'Anything that's keeping me alive: statins, blood thinners, pills for hypertension. Bin the lot. Make sure there's a DNR in place: I don't want to be brought back if nature steps in to carry me off,' he adds.

'We must tell the children,' I say.

'We must,' he agrees and squeezes my hand.

Chapter 10: A Silent Tsunami

How do you decide - once you understand your parent cannot take care of themself - which child will assume that care? Whose job is this? Do you list the pros and cons of one over another on a sheet of paper scored by neat columns? Who has more time, or works from home? Who lives in a house with fewer precipitous, unguarded stairs? Who has better services close by? Is it as cleanly incisive as that – as if in drawing up a table and checking boxes you'll calculate precisely the right place for them to be?

No: it can't be. It's an untidy sort of slow evolution as you tie up the raggedy ends and see which hold fastest. I am miles from a hospital. There are no care facilities near me. No health services to support. But I work for myself from home. I have sunshine, which means that sheets – and we must launder Mum's most days – dry fast as they flap cheerfully on the line and are crack-dry by noon.

And, I have help.

I imagine extra hands will mean if, when, Mum gets bad, I will have support to lift her in the absence of hoists or hospital beds. I imagine extra hands will give me a break when I become overwhelmed by all this. I imagine only the practical help of extra hands.

I have known Asina for over twenty years. She has lived with us for almost as long. Crucially, she has grown to know Mum, has borne witness to her extended visits. Neither speaks the other's language with any fluency but each makes herself understood and it is not long before Mum is insisting Asina stop and drink tea with her or 'Would you like a beer instead, Asina?' Asina, who even if she wasn't busy is a teetotal Muslim, howls with laughter and says tea is fine.

So, if I thought the support would be in stronger arms and somebody to help me bathe Mum or lift her from the loo, I was only half right. Yes, Asina saved my back. Yes, because there were always two of us, Mum was safe from falls in the shower even when slippery with suds.

But it was Asina's wise counsel that saved me most, her gentle insistence that looking after the elderly is what the young are supposed to do. When I grew frustrated, she would soothe, 'She's just old.' When I worried about the impact of all of this on all of us, she reminded me, 'But we must look after our mothers when they cannot look after themselves,' and I thought of her community of women – of mothers and nieces and sisters who rallied as a team around one another in her village. She never took offence at any of Mum's cross words: 'She doesn't mean it,' she laughed, so that I remembered this most personally insulting of illnesses is not personal. Asina and I knew one another so well that the shared intimacy of dealing with Mum's failing body – washing, toileting – became an exercise in pragmaticism. We each knew which bit of Mum to hold and how. The systems and routines we followed became instinctive.

In the beginning, Asina would tell me, 'Your mother is going to get well again,' and – after a really good day – 'See! She's much better already.'

I struggled to explain Mum's terminal diagnosis to her: 'She will not get better, Asina. She will only get worse.' Asina grew impatient with me then. Of course, she's getting better.

Couldn't I see the improvement in Mum: her appetite, the weight she was gaining?

Eventually I find an online leaflet in Kiswahili to describe the trajectory, and crucially, the prognosis of Dementia: *Kuelewa ugonjwa wa kupoteza fahamu* 'understanding the disease of unconsciousness' Google Translate helpfully provides.

Asina reads it and after that our conversations are about managing Mum today. That day. Our relationship becomes one of deep collaboration. Asina observes minute changes in Mum that I sometimes miss.

'What's this?' she asks and points to the first angry bloom of a pressure sore. I take a photo of Mum's hip and send it to my pharmacist who is in a town two hours' drive away. When, later in the week, I receive the medication he has prescribed, Asina and I apply it together and I sense her relief that she is doing something, anything, in the face of this illness I have told her there is nothing we can do anything about.

But, while we can see where pressure marks Mum's skin, what we cannot see – because Dementia, cruel artist of undoing, is startling both in its subtlety and its suddenness – is that this illness is not done yet. It is far from done. There is much more of Mum to undo, as if all of her DNA was a giant ball of colourful yarn, once neatly spooled, which Dementia is intent on pulling apart, an arm's length at a time.

When Mum first comes to live with me, she can dress herself, walk unaided, with just an unobtrusive hand beneath her elbow to prevent falls, guide her step. She can go to the loo on her own, accidents avoided thanks to pull-up diapers which she changes herself. She can butter her own toast, manage a knife and fork to cut up her own food and she eats with gusto.

A friend comes to visit four months after Mum arrives. She observes Mum, neatly dressed, hair brushed, flicking through a magazine while she sips a cup of tea. Mum, who looks normal, acknowledges her with a nod and a smile and a polite hello.

My friend's mother also has Dementia.

'But she's way worse than your mum, way, *way* worse. much more advanced (which is a strange choice of word given this is an illness about going backwards) your mum has a long way to go, a long, long way to go.'

And I am not reassured by this, not heartened by the fact Mum isn't as bad as she could be.

I am appalled at the thought that she will get worse.

Dementia is never as bad as you think it's going to be. Until it is. It keeps getting worse. Until it runs out of things to worsen.

⋆ ⋆ ⋆

Before Dementia revealed itself in my mother, I knew very little about it. And I did not seek to know much: I gave it a wide berth.

Another friend's mum suffered. And, for as long as she was able, my friend bravely dragged her mother everywhere, determined to keep her immersed in some extrinsic world. Her mother sat mute, eyes either vacant or wild, mostly avoided.

I gave *her* a wide berth too.

I don't have a choice now: now I am forced to face Dementia, to eat most of my meals in its company, to try to engage with it every day.

A lunchtime bowl of soup, which I would race through at my desk if I were on my own, turns into a tortuously slow affair when Mum's focus is on whatever it is we are eating.

'What's this?' she asks, peering into her bowl.

'Pumpkin soup,' I say.

'Gosh,' says Mum, 'I've never had this before,' as she brings a spoonful daintily to her mouth.

I made it with too much butter and just the right amount of cinnamon – more than the recipe said, always more – so the kitchen was scented, as the broth bubbled, with the sweet pepperiness of spice. I had inhaled and, as I stirred, a memory flared.

I am small. Seven or eight. My sister is a toddler on Mum's hip. We are making cinnamon toast for tea.

Mum toasts one side of slices of bread under the grill. Once done, she butters the untoasted sides and sprinkles them with sugar into which she's sifted just the right amount of cinnamon powder – more than the recipe said – so the sugar was dusted ochre. Then she puts them back under the eye-level grill so that we could watch the alchemy of sugar melting and browning right in front of us. Me and my brother, straining to see, on tiptoes, my little sister leaning forward watching the magic happen. And the kitchen was dense with sugar and spice and delicious anticipation. By the time we bit into the careful-it-might-still-be-hot toast, its caramel topping cracked like toffee.

With the withering of Mum's world, at first her interest in food – and by extension her appetite – expands to fill the gap.

'Look at the size of my tummy,' she would fret, patting it as – come to think of it – an expectant mum might her bump.

She develops an insatiable sweet tooth. When I try to understand why, I read that Alzheimer's causes a drop in insulin sensitivity which drives an appetite for sweet things. At the same time, Dementia is invading the prefrontal cortex – the brakes on the way we behave – so self-restraint goes.

Mum could eat a whole box of chocolates without apparently registering.

I wonder if our taste for sweet food is the last to go because it is the first to form in infancy. As if even that follows the bookshelf arc of Dementia. Breast milk is sweet, much sweeter than cows' milk. I know this from experience. Once, feeding one of my own babies at my breast, the other side began to leak. I had no cloth to staunch the flow so I used my hand to cup the drip-drip instead, and then – not knowing what to do with the pool collected in my palm – I licked it clean. I was astonished at its sugariness.

'What packet does the soup come from?' Mum wants to know.

'It's not from a packet Mum, it's homemade: pumpkin. From the garden'

'Oh.'

She isn't sure what a pumpkin is.

'It's a vegetable, Mum, a big orange one.'

Three minutes later: 'What is this we're eating?'

'Pumpkin soup.'

'It's very good,' she says.

I have to concentrate to respond with the same enthusiasm each time, so that I don't let a tone of irritation creep into my voice and betray my impatience: 'Isn't it?' I agree, for what feels like the tenth time in as many minutes.

There are many hard things about living with somebody with Dementia, many. One is the lack of a launch pad for conversation.

We cannot share our history anymore, and my mother cannot imagine a future. We live in the present, even when it's fabricated, as if spun from thin air. There is no continuum, no hooks to tether my stories to, no ballast to weight them, no anchors to ground them. Most of the time there's nothing. Where once we could gossip or giggle about friends and family, Mum remembers nobody; all the juicy bits squeezed dry by her Alzheimer's. Where once we could discuss the news she listened to as she drank morning tea in bed, we can't anymore. She cannot remember at breakfast-time which country is at war with which, or what despot is being ever more tyrannical. These things would once have driven lively, well-informed debate. Now we just float about the dining table, drifting from one element of the meal to another.

'This soup is delicious; what is it?'

In the absence of soup at breakfast time, it's the honey that takes centre stage.

'This jam is very good, did you make it?'

'It's honey, Mum – and no, the bees did.'

'Bees? Bees!'

Sometimes, and I am ashamed to admit it, to fill gaps, fast forward time, I resort to Wordle on my phone.

'Let's see if we can get today's word, Ma.'

She peers at my screen.

'On that?' And then, 'I've never played this before.'

I bite my tongue.

And I try – again – to explain the fundamentals of five letters, one word, what the green squares mean, why they're orange and how many attempts we're allowed. Mum looks on bewildered.

Mum who once tried to teach me how to do the cryptic crossword. Then it was my turn to look confused.

I complete the puzzle in the nick of time.

'Phew,' says Wordle.

'Look,' I say to Mum, 'We got it, we *just* got it.'

Note the 'We'.

I feel less guilty about playing a game on my phone to ease the tedium of lunch if I feign Mum's inclusion.

It's why, when something presents that prompts a recollection of my own, I grab it. Then I take my mother by the hand and lead her down memory lane to show her something we once did together.

'When we were small, you used to do this' and, with Mum watching intently, I pluck a segment of clementine from my plate. I split it down its seam with a fingernail and butterfly the citrus so its fleshy, tangerine innards are winged outwards.

'Oh yes,' says Mum, her expression lit, 'I remember!'

And there it is, a momentary flash: Something lost retrieved, something bright revealed, just like the inside of the piece of fruit she takes from me and pops into her mouth.

* * *

But later, on worse days, when Dementia steals my mother's grace and manners, when her illness has begun to reshape her face as a clumsy sculptor so that her eyes no longer dance with interest, so that their stasis steals into her expression and robs it of the lines that drew themselves as laughter, she morphs into some shouty monster whom I cannot please or placate.

This is this hideous anomaly of Dementia: when sufferers are at their most vulnerable, when they cannot climb steps alone or walk unaided because their shuffling gait means they are at risk of falls, when they are incontinent, cannot use a phone or the TV remote or shower without fear of slipping or scalding; when they would not eat if you did not put food in front of them, they can be bloody.

They can be really shitty.

'There was no hot water for my morning tea,' my mother proclaims imperiously when I stick my head around her door just after dawn, 'So I only had half a cold cup.' Her tone tells me this is my fault.

Once, on a better day, as Mum made a mug of tea for us both, she told me, 'I count the steps, there are four,' she said: 'hot water, tea bag, sugar, milk.' Except today there was no hot water, apparently.

'You must have finished all the water during the night, Mum,' I say – even though I urge her, every night, motioning to the clock, 'Don't get up until the big hand is on the twelve and little one on the 7.'

But Mum's concept of time is going the way of everything else.

'Sundowning' – that euphemistic phrase to describe the way Alzheimer's disease causes circadian rhythms to short-circuit so that the ends of the day are muddled and distressing – began to manifest in Mum weeks ago. 'Okay,' she might say, smiling obediently at my instruction to please not get up in the middle of the night. And then forgetting, so she is up at midnight, at 2 o'clock, Again at 4 o'clock. Drinking mug after mug of tea until the flask is drained.

Once upon a time, surfacing from episodes of Depression, drinking tea before sun-up would have heralded something hopeful – a reawakening in her, something emerging into the light after a long, dark hibernation, a can't-wait-for-the-day-to-begin optimism. Now it just means she doesn't understand what time of day it is.

* * *

I did not know that there was such a thing – but there is.

The writer, Dani Shapiro, describes this in her memoir, *Hourglass*.

When commissioned to write a play to foster empathy for Dementia sufferers, Shapiro and her husband attended a Virtual Dementia Tour where, to understand something of the plight of those living with Alzheimer's, they had to don scratched goggles, snap on huge headphones that played random noises into their ears – slamming doors, sirens, snatches of incomprehensible conversation. They had to wear several pairs of gloves which made them thick-thumbed, and shoes with sharp spikes built into the soles to create a similar sensation to the pin-pricking of neuropathy that plagues some sufferers of Alzheimer's. Shapiro wonders if that is why her mother-in-law shuffled. Thus burdened, these Dementia tourists were then obliged to carry out a number of simple tasks – sort pills, write a brief note, fold a blanket. Shapiro writes that she, like many others, gave up. 'It was just too hard,' she said.

I wander about the ether now, looking for a virtual simulation of my mother's devastation, trying to put myself in her shoes, which are described by the tour I find – and there are lots out there now – as being filled with stones: to mimic a precarious balance, the clumsiness of walking on marbles. Stones in your shoes, gloves filled with rice grains to affect the loss of dexterity, lenses over your eyes, smeared with Vaseline to cloud your vision.

In my imagination, thus hindered, half blind and hobbling, I am already shambling around, unable to walk with confidence, pick up a mug of tea and navigate it safely to my mouth without scalding or spilling. I can't see through the greasiness. And then a pair of headphones is slapped about my ears and filters a cacophony of senseless sounds into my head. I cannot concentrate on anything. I would not be able to complete a single one of the tasks – the writing of lists or sorting of laundry – without growing distracted.

Becoming, as one participant said, 'supremely frustrated.'

And in that frustration and confusion and distress and disorientation of my mother's world, and through the incessant hiss and rasp of unwelcome sound, there was I, the carer – insisting it was time for a shower or that my mother must finish her juice or go to the loo. Did my words pierce the dissonance and help bring her back briefly, steady her?

Or did they just add to the noise in her head?

* * *

Have you ever thought about how a memory forms? How it sticks, fast and firm, a limpet to a rock. I never did, not until I watched my mother's memories abandon her and then, I suppose, as in all I do now – that is, prophylactically – I sought to understand how I might secure my own.

I rolled the words around my mouth – amyloid plaques, tau tangles, amyloid plaques, tau tangles. As if in pinning them to memory, I was fastening a rabbit's foot to my collar to protect my own.

What makes a memory? What makes it stick? Which memories seed themselves deep and permanent in the structures of our brain? What feeds them so that they might germinate and take root, so that the memory sustains: a tiny acorn to a sturdy oak, growing branches of interconnectivity. Remember this? Remember that? Remember when? Remember them?

Memory, I learn, is uneven: not all memories are equal, they are cast of different beginnings – conscious and unconscious – and sculpted by different things. They can be stored in separate parts of the brain or several parts of the brain as each of those parts supplements and safeguards their storage. The brain's outer layer – the distinctive neocortex with its skin wrinkled like fingertips held underwater too long – supports the seahorse-shaped hippocampi by backing up our memories as we sleep. The corpus callosum – the brain's superhighway – is the route by which messages traffic between left and right hemispheres.

Memories, knowledge, emotion, behaviour and every single voluntary – walking, talking, eating – and involuntary – breathing, sneezing, salivating – action is the consequence of our finely tuned cerebral engineering. When it begins to stall, we do. It's why Dementia isn't just about forgetting.

But memory is where it begins. Some memories flit through, bright and brief, gossamer-winged as butterflies; they don't last: the minutiae of an ordinary day. Others sustain a lifetime: your parents, your partner, your children (until they don't). These long-lasting, firm-holding memories, the ones that require conscious retrieval – a reaching back and grasping hold of – are described as *explicit*. They can be episodic – when they are moulded out of experience – or semantic, when they relate to general knowledge.

The hippocampi are where episodic memories are formed, where new things that have been learned are reinforced as memory. They are the gateway to memory transfer – its first filing trays – and the lenses that remembers faces and places. I identify them on an image of the human brain now, this pair of sea-creature-curled vaults are deep in the temporal lobe.

Each component of the brain is spooned around another, like a nautilus. The basal ganglia, the metronome of habits formed, movement made, long-learned memories, like riding a bike, or swimming: I do not have to think about the strokes I make, the breaths I take, as I plough up and down a pool.

The hypothalamus – from the Ancient Greek *(hupó)* 'under', and θάλαμος *(thálamos)* 'inner chamber', to describe its position beneath the thalamus – directs the workings of our hormones, metabolism, body temperature, blood pressure, hunger, sleep, thirst. It drives a woman's maternal instinct.

I wonder, as I read this, if that was why my mother's invisible link to me became loosened? Because her hypothalamus grew starved and atrophied? It certainly explains why she began to complain of feeling cold despite the weight of so many blankets her skin was slick with sweat.

I trace the curl and folds of this shell-shaped organ as I map the different parts of it. I say their names out loud as if to paste them into my own memory: cerebellum, frontal and occipital lobes, medulla oblongata, cingulate gyrus, the almond-shaped amygdala which weights memories with emotional significance. I say them over and over as if reciting a poem.

And I think, as I roll the names of each around my mouth, that in the process I am cementing the episodic memory of my mother's Dementia as semantic in the facts and milestones of this devastating disease.

★

When my mother's memory first began to fail, I used to wonder how far back she had to stretch to retrieve some part of her past shape. And it seemed with every few months she had to reach further and further behind her. Dementia swept an eraser across the blackboard where my mother's story was written, and laid waste to it; We all became dust in the end.

All but her parents and one sister. They were the last standing, the heavy titles at the base of her bookshelf.

One evening as I tuck Mum up, careful to position her in the centre of her bed so there is less likelihood she will tip to the floor in sleep, as I arrange the accoutrements of night-time within arm's reach on her bedside table – specs, water in a child's sippy cup, a clock which will glow uselessly in the dark – I drop a kiss on my mother's head.

'Good night Mum,' she says with a sleepy smile, 'Say goodnight to Dad for me.'

For just a moment I feel winded. And I am reminded: Dementia is not a gentle slope to decrepitude. It is not the soft collapse of a cake taken out of an oven too soon so that it exhales itself to disappointing flatness. It is not the slow slide of a pat of butter as it melts. Dementia takes your breath away in bone-jarring steps – there's no time to acclimatise as you go down, down, down.

*

This is how I imagine my mother's brain. A sea sponge. Or a gouda cheese. The pockets of air between anything of substance are widening.

'The cortex shrinks where the cells used to be. The spaces in between expand. Islands in the sea of the mind. An archipelago of the former self,' wrote Sinéad Gleeson on Alzheimer's disease. And I think of my mother wading between these small landmasses in her mind where she can still find something solid of herself, and in between, where she drowns.

But, as I learn, again and again, Dementia is not just about memory, it is not just the falling away of our most recent histories. It is about the connections we once made, and now fail to, the language we loved and are losing, the personalities we were. And it is about shoring up the gaps that illness gouges with something that begins to look like madness.

('Why am I surprised?' I wonder, many months later, after all, think of the etymology of the word: Dementia.)

Mum is deeply distressed this morning. I find her outside in her bare-feet and nightgown. She is anxious to find her sister. Her parents.

Her room, when I lead her back, has been laid siege to. The cat has taken fright and long gone. The table fan is up-ended on the floor. There are books strewn and the bed is a tangle of sheets.

'Take it away,' Mum insists, 'take it away, that thing, maybe you need it.' The fan.

Beneath her bed I find tubes of cream, the alarm clock, her hairbrush.

She says it is time to go to bed.

It is 8am.

The day has already spun wildly out of control.

She is fretful and talks nonsense and takes empty mugs into the loo and cannot get her bearings anywhere.

I urge her to sit. I take a seat close to her. I hold her hand and she describes her night.

'I was out, at some place of entertainment. There were so many people there. I felt ashamed – I was only in my nightdress, you see. I don't think I knew anybody. I didn't know where you were. You were meant to be there but you were not. I got very tired but I couldn't find my way out. There was furniture all over the place. I wasn't able to climb over it to the door. I lay down eventually – on a bed or a table, I am not sure. I went to sleep.'

I tell myself: this must be what Dementia feels like: a maze.

Is this her imagination stuffing those ever-widening gaps in her brain, mortar in the cracks of a wall, lest the whole house come tumbling down? Do those with Dementia dream in psychedelic hues to colour a world that is growing greyer by the day? Is it fear?

The next day she has forgotten about this terrifying alien place she found herself wandering in, amongst strangers in her nightgown.

There it is again: the single generous thing about this dreadful disease – that she forgets her worst days – hours – fast.

Every day now, the memories I used to imagine Mum might still be able to grow, die faster. There's nothing to nurture them. They are shallow and weak and easily pulled.

How do I know?

Ten months after Mum comes to live with us, I am forced to make her a dentist appointment. A wobbly tooth has presented.

'It's sore,' she complains.

I administer painkillers but there are only so many days I can responsibly feed her ibuprofen before I understand that the inevitable cannot be put off; she needs to see a dentist.

I hate dragging Mum away from the sanctuary that home is, the place and people that live here, a tidy little organogram that lends context and construct to a coming-undone world. She might not know where we are (England, Ireland, Somewhere-in-Africa…). But mostly she knows she's At Home.

The morning dawns and Mum begins to articulate anxiety about our outing

'Am I making too much of a fuss?'

She doesn't wait for an answer: 'I think I'm making too much of a fuss.'

I know what she is doing: she is willing me to cancel, to call it all off. Leaving the safety of her bubble is frightening. *Where am I going? Who will we meet? Have I met them before?*

'We need to get this seen to, Mum,' I insist, 'Your tooth… while we can… while the dentist can see you,' before it flares into an infection I cannot manage with my sloppy over-the-counter approach.

'Yes, yes, you're right,' she agrees reluctantly.

Then, out of nowhere, 'He's not going to take a baby out, is he?'

'A baby…?'

And I am reminded of a rule I've recently made for myself: make no assumptions about Dementia. If I thought her anxiety was about leaving home, it might as easily have been because she has forgotten what dentists do.

'No, Ma,' and I can't resist a smile, 'Not a baby, maybe a tooth, the dentist might have to take the tooth out.'

Which is what he does. I primed him in my text message: *She has Alzheimer's.* He faces Mum and sweetly describes what he is going to do and why; he speaks to her as he might a child, he stoops to her level, and continues to reassure her as the back of the chair is lowered, checking she is comfortable.

Mum listens, her eyes round as the dentist explains that he will inject her gum to numb it first and then he will take the tooth out. I stand behind her, my hand on her shoulder so she senses my closeness.

She is baffled by the deadening sensation of gums: 'I can't feel my face,' she says, looking worried. I pat her gently, 'It's okay Mum, it's okay.'

She moans as the root is pulled. I am briefly alarmed. What if she doesn't understand we're trying to help and reacts to what must be painful and frightening, what if she lurches forward? But she doesn't; she just moans softly like something trapped and tired.

And then it's out and her mouth dribbles blood. Mum looks about her, dazed.

'All done,' we say, as if she were seven. As I have said to my own children before, 'All done.' And Mum gives us a little smile.

You don't think about taking Dementia patients to the dentist. You forget that in the falling apart of their cognition, their ailing, ageing physical selves have the propensity to fall apart too: joints, eyes, teeth, bladder, bowel. And you forget that in facing the enormous prognosis of Dementia, there are still the small everyday ailments that need addressing: a fungal infection between her toes, a sore throat, wax in her ears. A toothache. And these things are oddly comforting: small and ordinary, not catastrophic or terminal. I can make a difference to these.

When we get home, as soon as we get out of the car, Mum begins to fret, 'What is this place? Where are we? Why are we here?' Her face is creased by consternation.

'This is home, Ma,' I say, 'We left early this morning, for the dentist.'

(*Remember*?)

She won't have it. She grows agitated, she casts about herself as if she's left somebody behind or lost something important.

'And where are they?'

'Where is who?'

'***They***, them, ***them***,' she is almost hysterical: 'The people who lived here.'

'Me Ma, I lived – *live* – here. *With* you.'

'No,' she insists, 'No, no. Not you. They! ***Them!*** I can't believe they just upped and left without saying goodbye!'

'They didn't Mum, they – *we're* – still here.'

'What's your name?' she shoots.

'Anthea, Ma: I'm Anthea.'

'No, no, you're not,' cries Mum, 'You're not Anthea. Anthea's gone. I can't believe she left and never said goodbye.'

Dementia punctures memory so that our stories drip out. One by one, at first. Drip, drip. A dropped name, a lost event. A word. But with time, the disease rips those holes wide; the drip-drip of memory-loss becomes a stream, then a river, then a deluge and now the memories waterfall out. There is nothing left to hold them.

If I understand something of how memories form, I understand now how fast they can desert us: Within hours, my mother's are gone.

★ ★ ★

My husband is puzzled that I am compelled to remind my mother, again and again, that she has children, 'What's the point?' he asks.

'Because I want her to know she has family, who care, who will look after her,' I explain.

'Do you have children?' Mum asks politely.

'I do,' I say, 'Three.'

'How old are they?' she wants to know.

I tell her.

'About the same age as mine then, I suppose.'

'How many do you have?' I ask.

'Three. Or four,' she says.

'One died, when she was very little,' she states, without a trace of emotion: 'No idea why: she seemed perfectly healthy at the time.'

'Where *are* your children?' I sometimes ask.

She shrugs, 'Oh, I don't know – somewhere in Ireland, I suppose?'

Somewhere in Ireland. Somewhere in Africa. Somewhere, somewhere. Who knows?

We could be anywhere, for all she cares.

Sometimes I broach the fecklessness of these apparently unavailable children: 'Shouldn't they be looking after you?' I ask.

'I expect they're too busy,' she says, unfazed as she excuses the absence of this trio of errant progeny with a wave of her hand.

⋆ ⋆ ⋆

If I resist the word 'Depression' – too small, worn-out by overuse to convey the gravitas it should – I welcome the one that describes the undoing of my mother's cognition, her catastrophic forgetting so that even her children have been erased from her memories. We three go the way of lunch. We are lost to her along with the quiche and salad she ate with gusto and pronounced delicious at lunchtime, 'I've never had this before', only to tell me exactly the same thing when I produce the leftovers for supper.

If 'Depression' is too tame a word, too ambiguous, to capture the devastation, the alienation that accompanies melancholy, if it can just as easily be applied to weather fronts and economic collapse as the fragmentation of soul and psyche, 'Dementia' is not.

If Depression seemed like the arrival of a stranger, Dementia is the perpetual leaving of somebody you love; it is a thinning of everything that was Mum. She is in there, hidden beneath layers of lost memories like dust or ash. But sometimes, very rarely now, something will propel her old self forward and she will startle me with a word or a name from the past that pops up sharp and accurate and sudden.

'Tita,' she calls me one night, 'Tita.' My childhood nickname. She does not remember I am her daughter most days and yet there it is: a familial moniker. I am as surprised as she is. It's like turning over old soil and unearthing a forgotten daffodil bulb ready to explode to sunny brightness.

And humour. That is another curiosity of all this: The humour that occasionally accompanies Dementia and never came, of course, (for that would be oxymoronic) with Depression.

My mother sometimes laughs easily, a rich glorious laugh that folds her face into creases so that it looks rounder and fuller and flushed, and she looks younger.

'Where's my helmet?' she demands as she steps into the shower.

'You mean your shower cap?'

And we both surrender to a fit of giggles.

Or when she readies herself in the morning: up, dressed, hair brushed, shoes and socks on.

'Ready,' she announces.

'And your teeth?' I ask.

And she gives me the broadest, gummiest grin, 'My teeth! I knew I'd forgotten something!'

She has forgotten a lot. But I don't say that. I just laugh: 'Your teeth,' I confirm.

Standing upright on the shores of health or youth, our feet

rooted in the sand, our balance and perspective safe and steady, we are all staring out into a dark and forbidding sea where there is a wave, cresting white headed and thunderous: a silver tsunami. That's what it's called: this rising tide of Dementia sufferers. We don't see it until it washes over us. Still Alice wasn't still Alice at all. My mother is no longer my mother.

But even if our awareness of the word, the illness, is being sharpened, it is happening too slowly. Dementia is not new: it's as old as melancholy. The word is pasted through language, has cemented itself – a plaque – to every century. From the Latin *demens*, 'out of one's mind', it existed in sixteenth-century English, *demency*, and French, *démence*. As far back as Homer's *Odyssey* – in the eighth century BC – there is reference to this memory-stealing disease.

As a young man, King Laertes of Ithaca was an heroic figure. When his son, Odysseus, disappeared to fight the Trojan War, King Laertes receded from court, wore rags instead of robes. He grew disconnected from royal life and preoccupied himself with his garden and his animals instead.

When Odysseus returns and explains his absence, describes his adventures to his father, 'a dark cloud of sorrow fell upon Laertes as he listened. He filled both hands with the dust from the ground and poured it over his grey head, groaning'. He does not recognise his son.

'If you really are my son Odysseus,' Laertes begged, 'you must give me such manifest proof of your identity as shall convince me.'

'First observe this scar,' answered Odysseus, 'which I got from a boar's tusk when I was hunting.'

Then he walks his father through the orchard, 'I will point out to you the trees you gave me,' he said, 'I asked you all about them as I followed you round the garden. You told me their names. You gave me thirteen pear trees, ten apple trees and forty fig trees.'

I have witnessed Laertes' distress in my mother, watched that same 'Are they lying to me?' confusion fog her expression. I have felt Odysseus' anguish; I know his determination to prove who he is to his father.

In the Middle Ages the forgetting that attended Dementia was believed to hold up your passage to heaven. Or hell. Your 'forgetting' rendered you an unreliable witness: how *could* you tell the difference between right and wrong? And I think: aren't they there already – these victims of that wave, their memories all drowned out? Or is my mother on some godforsaken raft in Limbo – with no land in sight to orient her? How could you argue a seat in paradise if you couldn't remember whether you'd been good or bad? (And I vow to send my mother with a note for St Peter when she is dispatched. It will say, 'Don't hold her up at the Pearly Gates; I can vouch for her: a person of deep faith, a well of goodness.')

The thirteenth-century doctor, Roger Bacon, wrote, 'senility is a consequence of the original sin.' And I think I shall add a postscript in my note to St Peter: 'Born to good Catholic parents, my mother was baptised at three weeks' old in a church in Bombay' – and I'll send the certificate with her for good measure.

I show my mother my own metaphorical scars now. I take her hand and walk her through figurative orchards. I plant photograph albums around Mum's chair, her bed, on every surface, the oldest I can find.

1964.

She recognises my father in every single picture, my young, handsome father, 'There's Jim!' she says and relief floods her face: there is her life. It is still here.

★

Not everybody would agree with me that 'Dementia' is the right word for this disease. Within the last decade doctors and scientists have posited that we need one that is less pejorative, more meaningful. They suggested 'frontotemporal disease' in its stead.

What if you do not know what part of a body that alludes to? Or which vital part of a person it steals? (All of them, as it turns out; it has ransacked my mother.)

No, I prefer 'Dementia'. There is no doubting with 'Dementia'. It's a hard, cruel, unambiguous word.

★

But Dementia, even if it is the right word, is not linear. It is not the opposite of a negative being exposed; Dementia is not its back-to-black reverse. Dementia is not like watching a person fade with the twilight until the night has swallowed them up. Dementia is like being on a stage beneath strobe lights: sometimes elements are sunk into blackness and sometimes they are illuminated with brilliant and shocking brightness. They come and they go until they are gone.

One day my mother knows precisely who I am.

Anthea. You are ***that*** *Anthea.*

The next: nothing.

Who are you anyway?

One day she knows precisely who my sister is: who she is to her, to me, how to pick her out of the tatty line up on my fridge whose steely exterior is humanised with a hundred smiling faces, old and young. The next, she has died. *No idea why.*

And I think it is this, this patchiness, this-sometimes-she'll-know-me and sometimes-she-won't that make Dementia harder to acclimatise to: it's a rollercoaster of soaring highs when a small hopeful kernel of memory rises to the surface. And crashing lows.

My husband's advice is to roll with the punches. And he is right: get your balance, steady yourself, catch your breath between blows. Mum cannot remember the bruisings her illness rains on the rest of us. She does not feel any residual ache – and I am glad.

Mum will argue with me and argue with me until I relent: 'Yup, you're right Ma: we came here by boat' (Here: to my mountainous landlocked corner of northern Tanzania) because she refuses to accept we are not docked in some exotic port. And because of this conviction, that we are surrounded by sea, she will be loath to step into the garden in case she drowns.

She will pack her suitcase two mornings in a row at 4am because she insists I told her we will set sail at dawn. I will bring her tea and find her up and dressed and ready to go. She will motion to the belongings she is leaving behind: 'These things: they are not mine,' she will announce and I will see amongst them the blouse she wore two days ago.

It is better, I find, to be frank about Dementia. That way, nobody is shocked by the inconsistencies that present in Mum, nobody will say, 'Oh but we've met before.' And so she will be spared some small embarrassment, the conflict of not knowing something everybody else does. Because everybody will play along with this charade and everybody will play their part in the casting and recasting of flimsy memories. Every single time my friend Eliza visits, and she visits often, she bends low over Mum and takes her by the hand. 'Hello,' she smiles, 'I'm not sure we've ever met, I'm Eliza.' And Mum beams up at her.

And I think that's the way it's done: the frank introduction of this thing that nobody wants to name.

★

But if Dementia is the right word, 'carer' isn't. I take issue with its soft sound, delivered in rounded letters and purred syllables. 'Carer' doesn't describe me. It only describes – some of – what I do. And 'carer' conjures something of the saint I am not, 'You're quite prickly at times, you know,' says a friend. And I bristle.

I prefer to think of myself as my mother's minder – for that word – *minder* – conjures some small part of the muscle and the advocacy we must exercise as the soft-sided carers we are not; it summons something of the bounce and the bouncer.

Roll with the punches.

If asked, in that role, what small wisdom I could impart, what shard of clear-eyed insight on how to handle the day to day of this devastating die-a-thousand-deaths disease, what would I offer?

I'd say: Smile. Smile because if you do, the whole world smiles with you? (Cry and you cry alone?) No, nonsense platitudes have no place here – they don't have the spine to stand up to all this. No, you must smile, one of the geriatricians I spoke to told me, because it will help the person who birthed you and raised you trust the stranger you have become. If Mum trusts me, she will oblige me: in changing her clothes, putting on her shoes, coming for a walk, opening her mouth to another spoon of Weetabix. And, if I smile at her, she will smile back at me. And then – briefly – she is whole: her smile plumps a face made gaunt by this disease, lights eyes dimmed by it. And so then, for an instant, her old well self trips across her expression. And it is easier to do this job when I see my mother return fleetingly.

Touch them, I'd say. I scrub Mum's back in the shower as rivulets of hot water trace the curl of it, I wield a flannel until it lathers. Afterwards, having manoeuvred her towards a chair so that she can sit, I towel her vigorously, rubbing pale skin until it blushes. I sit on the floor and cradle her feet in my lap, I dry between each toe. She responds with oohs of pleasure or giggles, 'That tickles.' When I wash her hair, I knead her skull beneath my fingertips as if I could reshape the broken bits.

I will worry later – did I touch her enough? Touch in affection, not just ablution?

Record yourself when in conversation with the person you're 'minding'. It is weeks too late that I find a voice note on my phone where I captured a conversation between Mum and me. I think I taped it to try to convey something of her fast unravelling to my siblings. Did I ever send it to them? Did I even listen to it myself? I listen to it now. I hear Mum's anxiety about where her money is, who has taken all her money, what will she do without it. I hear my short – even sharp – replies, 'Your money is safe. Nobody stole it. Stop worrying about money.'

I hear my excuses now: I was tired. I was frustrated by the stuck-record-fretting, a needle scratch-screech, over and over. I had things to do.

I want to erase the conversation. I want to have it again, but differently. I want to smooth my words with patience, soften my tone, lower my pitch. Perhaps even present my mother with a purse full of coins for her to inspect and tuck into her dressing gown pocket. I told myself I'd buy into the fiction to disguise the fact. I want to rewind and play it all over again.

It's too late. I don't erase the recording: a reminder. Be kinder.

⋆ ⋆ ⋆

Hat says to me on a walk, a late evening walk, so late I must push my sunglasses to the top of my head for the last of the afternoon is tipping over my western horizon and the sharp edges of daylight are smudged by a buttery gloaming, 'I hope you don't get what Gran has.'

What Gran Has.

And then she asks, 'What do you do, Mum, to make sure you don't get it?'

What do I do?

What *can* I do?

What *should* I do?

I notice every article about Dementia. That's what I do. They leap from the page, from a screen, like wagging fingers.

5 Ways to Prevent Alzheimer's, Says Dr Sanjay Gupta

Keep moving, eat a healthy diet, avoid sugar, get enough sleep, be social. If it were only that simple.

I, who sits at my desk too long, too often a mug of sweet tea at my side, to give me a boost after a bad night, to sustain me through an afternoon when I'd like to nap but need to write.

I, the introvert.

Can I strike these habits out with others? Create a mitigating balance? If I walk enough – five miles a day, fast, so that my heart pounds and my breath comes short and sharp, so that I can still talk but cannot sing – will that temper the dangers of the writer's necessarily sedentary life? If I rarely eat meat, pile my plate high with organic veg, will that make up for sugar in my tea, frequent squares of chocolate? If I hold more conversations in the ether than I do in real life as I interview doctors and scientists all over the world in my job as a journalist, will that counteract my lonely, remote living?

Can I make extenuating trades?

Later, and with our conversation still fresh in my mind, I can feel Hat's eyes on me as we watch *The Father* on television.

Anthony Hopkins shuffles in and out of subtly changing rooms which morph from dark wood Sixties' decor to bright contemporary sleek. He is mostly bewildered, often belligerent, always paranoid ('Where is my watch? Who stole my watch?') and frequently in his pyjamas. Occasionally his words are shot with brilliant, sharp lucidity. Often they are acerbic, even cruel. Sometimes his observations, his recollections (which baffle his daughter) are funny.

I am at the tail end of a head cold. When I sniff, Hattie shoots me a sidelong look, I smile to reassure her.

I watch and I immerse myself in Hopkins' world, one of disorientation, in this shapeshifting environment where corridors widen and narrow so that doors which lead to one room in one scene lead to quite another in the next. And where people are sometimes two-faced: so that his daughter presents as her older, then her younger, and then again her older self and where he insists a new carer is his other, younger daughter.

Once I might have been disorientated in Hopkins' world. Not now: now I find myself in his lost rooms.

'Where is she *anyway*?' Hopkins asks of his daughter.

('Anyway'. A word I hear my mother use a lot now: a tool to minimise the enormity of all this – as if the question doesn't matter – 'Who are you *anyway*?')

She is dead. But this memory eludes him.

He fills the tragic gap with a stuffing of fabrication that I recognise: she is travelling. His lost daughter. She is away. She is a painter.

My husband left me, you know.

How can you forget your child is dead?

But you can.

How can you forget your own daughter?

But Mum has.

I am struck that art can deliver such a profound portrayal of an illness that is all about forgetting and fraying, that a screenplay has spun all of this together and has delivered a story I recognise so well. In Olivia Colman as Hopkins' daughter, I see myself. There is something reassuring in her delivery: the unmooring of my mother is manifest in millions of people. And so too are my reactions to it: the humour, the frustration, the rage, the sadness. I feel less alone as I watch. And I feel vindicated in the messy emotions I struggle to manage.

I do not shed a single tear until the very end when Hopkins says, as he weeps, 'I feel as if I am losing all my leaves.'

For he has articulated what my mother cannot: that she is shedding parts of herself, all of her selves have come undone and disappeared until all that is left is some unrecognisable skeleton in this dark wintering of her life.

Feathers for leaves.

I cry then.

★ ★ ★

I am fascinated by the fiction my mother spins during our conversations. Not just the big fictitious conclusions she comes to because what else could possibly explain my father's absence – *He just upped and left me* – but the small apparently inconsequential: the fattening of conversation starved by Dementia.

She colours her stories with great detail: She will explain a thing thus, 'She made a telephone call, you see,' or 'He could not drive himself; his car was broken down, you understand.' These fabrications are textured with the minutiae we all use to breathe life into anecdotes. She weaves the particulars together, I notice, to bring some fluency to the telling. It is as if the substance of those stories has gone but some knowledge of the craft of storytelling sustains.

Sometimes I love that she patches all the holes up with make-believe, as if dragging the seams of her coming-undone life together with untidy stitches.

We are watching a documentary about the Queen in the days after Her Majesty's death. Mum is riveted. Not everything on the television captures her attention but this does. I watch her face as she watches the screen and she begins to comment: 'I had no idea.'

She says it again, 'I simply had no idea.'

When she exclaims about having 'no idea' for the third time, I ask her: 'About what, Mum? What did you have no idea about?'

'I had no idea she was so famous. Mum and Dad never mentioned it.'

I am puzzled: 'Why would they though, Mum?'

Mum stops looking at the television and looks at me

instead, 'Because she used to stay with us all the time! All the time!'

I stifle a small laugh, 'How amazing,' I say.

'Yes,' says Mum, looking smug at the thought she knew somebody so famous, 'Yes, it is, isn't it?'

Mostly now, I do not correct her. I let her tell her stories. I ask questions to prompt her. To feign conviction or interest. Sometimes her tales take me to surprising places – HRH, a regular visitor in her parents' home – and sometimes it's exactly that which makes them so marvellous. Sometimes I laugh out loud and say, 'Oh Ma – I never know where we're going to end up when you tell a story, a whistle stop tour of the world!' (as we ricochet between India and Ireland and Africa as if all these places could be visited – for real – between lunch and supper).

And she laughs too.

When I ask questions, though, I wonder, feeling guilty, should I be doing this? Looking for things that are not there? Am I conspiring? Being condescending? Am I de-robing a naked emperor of still more invisible clothes?

But one morning when I call into her room to see how she slept, I find her up and drinking tea and dressed in something odd and mismatched. I say she must be cold. She ignores me. She is very agitated. She has been up for hours. I saw her light on at 4 o'clock in the morning. (But I didn't have the strength to investigate that early.)

'Who moved all my stuff in here?'

I look blank.

'Well?' she demands again, 'Who moved all my things – *all* my things – from my room to this,' she waves her hands around, 'to this new place?'

'I tried to get you on the telephone' she says, gesturing to the remote control, 'to ask where you were, where I was, but I couldn't get you.'

Some fiction I can buy into. Some I cannot.

'Nobody moved your stuff, Ma, this is your room, your space, these are all your things.'

And I think of the shoemakers' elves, I think of them sewing boots and slippers together at night, in the dark with even stitches and sturdy thread and concentrated industry, I think of them leaving them lined in tidy rows on the cobbler's workbench for him and his wife to find in the morning. And I think, Dementia does the very opposite: it is as if, as she slept, some unseen thing took a pair of tailor's scissors to her cognition and sliced through her thoughts and her recollections and all the things that still made a little bit of sense, so that whatever bits of her memory held the shape of her life together yesterday are in tatters this morning.

I am struggling with a response. I try to reason with her.

Mum's tone rises and she is firm, 'Oh come on. I am NOT stupid! I know, I KNOW, somebody moved all these things during the night. Even my bedclothes, *even* my bedclothes have been moved and dumped on this new bed.'

The one she slept in, the bed she climbed into last night when she knew where she was. The bed she sleeps in every night. Has slept in for over a year.

Diversion is a useful tool, it is a tactic I harness often now: 'Come Mum, let's go and have breakfast.'

'Where?' She wants to know. 'Where?'

'In the dining room,' I say.

I hope the excitement of tea and toast (when she will remark as she did yesterday and the day before that and all the days before that, how delicious the marmalade is and did

I make it and how much she loves the bread here and can she save her crusts for the dog) will distract her.

It does not. She prattles on and on and on about where she found herself in the night and how she wanted to escape and how all her things had been moved and how she could not get out because somebody had locked her door.

Finally I ask, 'Were you scared, Mum? To find yourself in a strange place?'

And there I am again: endorsing this invention, this stuff of make-up and madness.

'Well yes I was, I was afraid I might fall into one of the holes.'

One of the holes.

* * *

When Alan Bennett wrote about his mother in his *Untold Stories*, he described her hanging onto her handbag – clutching it even as an in-patient in hospital, stuffing it under her pillow for safekeeping 'as if she were in a strange and dangerous hotel'.

Her bag is an anchor. Something tangible to tether her to her old self. Something pitiful but patent grounding her.

I think of this every morning when I see my mother, her diary firmly in hand.

Since the beginning of the year, when the diary was new, she has announced, 'I must write in my diary today.' She says it every day. Sometimes she checks the date with me. Or the day of the week. Even the month.

'Gosh. Are you sure? April already?'

We identify the right date and Mum smooths the pages with a flattened palm.

'I'll write in it today.'

There is a single entry in the diary: 'I am in Ireland.'

She wasn't. She was – is – in Africa.

Mum used to keep a diary. Long ago she shared entries with me, entries that described her collapse into melancholy, her soaring flights from the depths of Depression. Her sickness. Her wellness. The advice of doctors, the encouragement of Catholic nuns. Lists of resolutions.

Get up early

Walk every day

Learn to say No

If only she had.

Her diary now, the one she never writes in despite telling me – and herself – every morning at breakfast time that she is going to do just that, is neither a place of wellness nor sickness.

It is simply a marker of time.

A place to count off the days.

Almost all the pages are empty.

Only my mother is written within that barrenness.

Chapter 11: Drowning not Waving

Sometimes it feels as if Alzheimer's has peeled off the layer that kept my mother's manners in place.

A band-aid of inhibition lies curled in the dust at our feet.

My mother would never have said the things she sometimes says now, have done the things she sometimes does. She would have recoiled from such behaviour.

She lifts a piece of bread high above her plate at breakfast time and drops it.

'Mum!'

'It's stale,' she sneers, 'Look.' And she moves to repeat the exercise by way of demonstration.

'Fine,' I snap. 'Don't eat it then.'

Or, 'My supper is horrid.'

(Of the lasagne she loved last week.)

Or, 'This programme is stupid.'

(Of the show she enjoyed so much yesterday, she watched it three times.)

She is not telling me these things conversationally. She is complaining.

And then: 'Sorry if you made it,' of the lasagne, not sounding in the least bit sorry.

Some mornings, resistant to rising, she rails against my – equally stubborn – resistance to her lying in bed all day.

Some mornings I have to drag her from her bed, lead her, like a recalcitrant old dog at the end of a taut leash, to the loo so we can change her diaper. And all the while she keeps up a litany of woes: 'I don't want to get up, why do I have to get up? I want to stay in bed.'

'You need to get up, Mum, because I need to help you change, I need you to drink, I need you to eat.'

'And then I need to go to work,' I say. (It is almost ten. I have achieved nothing for days.)

'Oh I see,' she hisses, 'It's all right for you: I have to get up only for you to abandon me and go to work.'

I see nothing of my mother here this morning. I cast about the room and look for her. But no, she's left for the day. Her sweetness replaced by rancour. Her solicitude by self-centredness.

This feature of Dementia, this peeling of that skin happens, I read, because of a thinning of cortical thickness in the right frontal lobe of the brain.

There are cerebral reasons to explain every new manifestation of Dementia – the lack of balance, the dropped words, the incontinence, the so-called 'sundowning' – and now the disinhibition. And it helps to track them – as if in tracking the reasons why they happen, I can keep track of the person my mother was once. And to know the physiological reason for the changes in the way Mum behaves reminds me to try to be patient.

Disinhibition is common, says the neuropsychologist I speak to – and it's another thing that those who look after people with Dementia are often unprepared for, she adds. She likens it to being drunk: 'When somebody has had a few drinks, the frontal lobe does not function as well as it would normally, so people say and do things that are out of character. This is a part of the brain that is affected by Dementia so naturally the functions of that area are disrupted.'

My well mother, a thin shadow increasingly eclipsed by the growing profile of my sick one, is in a constant futile tussle to reassert her old self, as if scooping bits of herself together, picking up those old band-aids, scraping the dirt off and reapplying them. But they never stay put.

★ ★ ★

'Why do you think she walks like that – without picking her feet up?' I ask my sister.

'Because she's afraid she'll fall?' my sister offers.

She is partly right; the trademark Dementia-shuffle happens because of a complex interplay of changes in the brain. As the disease gathers momentum, so sufferers slow their pace, shorten their slide, fold towards the ground for fear of losing balance. These changes are subtle to start with – in the same way the disease insidiously slinks into conversation – *leaves for feathers* – so it creeps into the way sufferers move. Scientists, using special devices, can detect early evidence of changed gait long before it is witnessed by the naked, uneducated eye in 'curve walking'.

Curve walking is just that – walking a non-linear path, rounding a bend, navigating any course that isn't straight. Curve walking demands better balance, coordination and cognitive planning than walking a straight line: Dementia settles into the corners first, I find.

As Mum's disease advances, she forgets what to do with her feet once she's standing. I haul her up and then remind her, when she asks, in bewilderment, 'What do I do now?'

'One foot in front of the other, Ma,' I say, and I tug her trouser leg at shin-level as a prompt.

'Oh yes,' she says and shuffles a foot forward.

One foot in front of the other.

Sometimes I tell myself the same thing.

★

Mum begins to complain, 'These slippers make my feet go like this,' and – because the language to describe this eludes her now – she shows me, from her seated position, how her soles slide when she tries to stand up. My sister and I source a pair of Dementia-friendly slippers on Amazon, then.

And I hate them. They feel like an admission. A giving in to this illness. A giving up in the face of it.

(Who am I kidding: Dementia always wins in the end.)

And the phrase, the jargon: Dementia-*friendly*.

What could possibly be 'friendly' about this horrible disease?

★

I have to prompt Mum to drink. Every day. All day. If I didn't, she never would.

'Here Mum,' I say, nudging a glass in her direction, 'Have some juice?'

I conjure all kinds of tricks to try to make her drink. On bad days I mix Coca Cola with water. For a bit, her sweet tooth is what chases the drink down. Not thirst.

'Do you think she doesn't get thirsty anymore?' I ask my sister.

She doesn't know, so we ask Google: *in Alzheimer's the centres in the brain that correspond to thirst stop working.* Which explains why Mum never, *ever* (not on a hot day) reaches voluntarily for a glass of water. But this necessary task, 'Drink, Ma, drink,' the relentless bid to keep her hydrated exacerbates her incontinence.

Why doesn't she know when to go?

A dribble becomes a deluge, and the odd pair of wet pants turns into bin bags full of adult diapers.

Later, when Mum's appetite begins to drop off, I spend hours trying to coax food into her: soup made with leeks and parsley for iron and fortified by the patience I'll need when I feed it to her.

'I don't like this.'

This is too salty.

This is too cold.

This is too hot.

The grisliest of Goldilocks and the Three Bears.

This is horrid.

Nothing is ever Just Right.

'Try it,' I beseech, in a voice you'd use with a stubborn toddler as you hold a spoon, animated as an aeroplane, in front of pursed lips.

And briefly, a memory, my memory (*of course* it's mine): My mother reading Dr Seuss's *Green Eggs and Ham* to my fussy younger brother, 'You *do* not like them, so you say! Try them! *Try* them! And you may.'

Where did the appetite go? Did taste take it when it abandoned her?

Taste changes affect seventy per cent of those with Dementia. The distortion – and sometimes abandonment – of taste worsens as the disease progresses. A disease eating your brain so you lose the interest – instinct – to feed yourself. It seemed crueller, when I got used to it, than my mother forgetting I was her daughter (after all, she needed to eat more than she needed to know who I was).

'This food tastes delaminated,' Mum says, wrinkling her nose and pushing her plate away.

Delaminated?

Taste perception is managed by the gustatory cortex, the bit of the brain in charge of processing signals from the taste buds. In Dementia, because there is a progressive atrophy of brain cells, those of the gustatory cortex follow the terminal pattern of deterioration. As a result, the ability to perceive different tastes is muddled and muddied; what might have been too salty grows unbearably bland.

'This tastes of absolutely nothing,' Mum grimaces, dropping her fork into a plate of fish pie.

Imagine that fundamental sense so bent out of shape, you no longer enjoy the taste of chocolate because the sweetness is bitter on your tongue, no longer relish the piquancy of the strong cheese you've always loved, (*This tastes of sand*); the last morsels of life's pleasures stolen from you.

And as 'carers', if we cannot even nourish those in our charge, what good are we?

'This,' Mum says, pushing a bowl of cereal away from her, 'has absolutely *nothing* to do with me.'

'You must eat SOMETHING, Mum,' I beg, trying to keep my voice even.

She regards me for a moment and then lifts her hand to her mouth and mimes the action of chewing her nails.

'That's not funny,' I say (though secretly I am admiring of this quick-witted response to my nagging).

'I am full,' she announces, her hand over her mouth so I can't get my airborne spoon into it, 'I made my own soup earlier. I ate that,' says my mother who has not cooked in years, who could not stand in a kitchen to prepare anything, no matter how 'Dementia-friendly' the lighting, the apparatus, the bloody slippers she stood up in.

* * *

Dementia, I have observed, carves the world up, cleaving continents and countries apart and rearranging them chaotically as if to mimic the cerebral mayhem that caused all this in the first place: the world does not look like the world anymore.

First my mother lost the names of countries.

It's just your stroke, I said to Mum.

Pure Alexia, I said to friends, as if knowing the name of the diagnosis meant I knew what I was talking about. (*She's lost everything with a capital letter, the names of all the people and all the places.*)

So first it was forgotten countries. And then it was where those countries were. As if somebody had spliced a map of the world up, into jigsaw pieces and put them all back together again in the wrong place so that our map looks like a globe made of Picasso-parts.

Then she lost the polar frame of reference for North and South. She cannot understand why my brother, in Ireland, is not experiencing the same broiling February weather we, in the summertime Sub-Saharan south, are complaining about.

'But it's so hot,' she says, peering at him on Skype, fanning herself with a book, 'Don't you think?'

And then the context of all the countries goes: what happened when and to who and where. As if her fragmented memories and flawed reasoning must scramble between what's left so they find themselves crowded together in the one place. It's like watching a motley collection of survivors from a shipwreck crawl ashore the same tiny island in the middle of a vast, deep sea, whose sandy sides are licked away with every tide.

And so Mum's known places, those refuges of safe harbour, that familiar geography is nibbled away and nibbled away until all that remains is the spot where she is sitting now.

And then even those parts get moved around in her mind:

'Where is my bedroom?'

'Where is my bathroom?'

'But that's not where I slept yesterday.'

'It's where you'll sleep tonight, Mum. It's your new room. Do you like it?' I ask, when I feel strong, 'Here, let me show you around,' as I take her hand and lead her from where she is sitting through the door that links to her bedroom where I point out the photographs beside her bed, her talcum powder (which grounds her more than the image of my father), her dressing gown. And from there to her bathroom, 'See? Your shower cap,' I say.

But sometimes, when I've had enough of Dementia, I don't have the energy for guided tours and so on those days, I sigh, 'Mum, it *is* your room, you slept here last night and the one before that and before that and all the nights before that.'

★

My mother's anxiety this evening is drawn on her face. Her eyes are wide and watching, her gaze follows me about the room as I ready it for the evening, closing windows, drawing curtains, cues to prod her primal parts, her animal physiology to know: *nearly bedtime, Mum.*

I sit down opposite her.

'Are you all right, Mum?'

'I am worried.'

'Why are you worried, Mum?'

She cannot find the words anymore – this woman, who was once so articulate. She cannot navigate language to describe why she feels the way she does. I must grope my way about her mind instead, look for lost things in the dark, try to locate fragments of those feelings, piece them together, and attempt to fathom the anxieties she is unable to voice.

Often now she threads the air with her fingers as if she might catch lost words like butterflies.

'Are you happy?' I prompt.

'I'm not sure.'

'Do you like living here?' I ask.

(Wherever here is).

'I do,' she says, 'very much.'

I ask her if she likes the garden, her room, *this* room, visits from the cat, short walks with the dog.

'I do,' she says, 'I do.'

'In that case, I think you should live here forever, with me, for the rest of your days, in this home, what do you think?'

I think she might cry. Relief floods her face, 'Oh, that would be too, too wonderful! Are you sure?'

'Of course I'm sure, we would love you to live here, with us.'

'Oh, thank you. Thank you.'

And so I learn that my mother does not feel safe unless I remind her that she is.

'Who trained you to do this?' she asks one day

'Do what?'

'Look after people.'

'I learned from my mother.'

Mum considers my words for a moment and then, 'She must have been a very kind woman.'

'She was,' I smile, 'I was very lucky.'

'And I am too,' she says, 'And now that I'm staying, I shall so look forward to getting to know you.'

* * *

And then Mum begins to tell me she sees things that are not there.

Faces at the window, children on the lawn, a man in the garden.

'Who do those children belong to?' she asks, pointing outside.

The first time I hear her asking, I follow the direction of her finger. As if there really might be somebody there and I am puzzled when there isn't.

My husband, who often sits reading close to where Mum sits pretending to, says, in an even, unsurprised tone, 'Just the neighbours.'

'And that man with them?' Mum presses, sounding anxious.

My husband cranes his neck as if to get a better look, 'Oh, I think that's their dad – he's very patient with them, isn't he?'

Mum sinks back into her seat and smiles, still watching, but relaxed now, 'Yes, he is,' she observes.

I will ask my husband afterwards how he knew to respond – for I will learn later that he did exactly the right thing: calmly bought into the fiction: of course there was nobody there.

He shrugs, 'Well no point arguing, is there?'

This is not the same as the fiction Mum has stuffed conversational gaps with, the skewed facts fattened to fill holes, like the little exaggerations you might overlook when a gifted raconteur is telling a story. Little bits of colour to brighten the boring bits, literary licence. This is Mum moving from the pockmarked place she inhabits to some entirely alternate reality.

★

One day, a friend, Marieke, who is a neurologist, comes to visit – ostensibly to have lunch with us. But covertly to observe Mum: the way she moves, eats, talks, responds.

'Could you just have a look at her?,' I had asked, 'Help me understand?'

Over lunch of soup and salad, ('Watch her when she eats,' Marieke will warn later, 'She's aspirating') Mum tells her about India. She tells her about her father who was a doctor. She tells her about her childhood in Africa. It is not seamless, but the threads of her story are just holding it together. Marieke looks at me from time to time and I furtively nod assent.

My father was a doctor. I used to live in Tanganyika. I was born in Bombay.

(And I think: old names, old maps).

In the middle of lunch, Mum gestures to the window, her brow crosshatched with concern,

'There are two people there, see, what are they looking at, what do they want?'

Marieke looks at me.

'They'll go just now, Mum,' I say, 'Not to worry.'

Later, with Mum tucked up in an armchair for a siesta, a blanket pulled up to her chin, Marieke wants to understand something of my mother's past. I describe serious and enduring psychiatric illness, I describe my father's death, I tell her about Mum's stroke and her loss of reading.

She says Mum's life sounds traumatic. She says such trauma can leave scars.

Marieke is a doctor with four degrees. She has a lot of knowledge to impart – my mother's illness is advanced, she says (and something in the word shocks me: *advanced*) evidenced, she explains, by Mum's gait.

Then she says, 'How often do they happen? The hallucinations?'

And there we have it: terrifying confirmation that things really are getting worse. I tell her Mum sees people in the garden. I tell her she sees them there often now.

When Marieke leaves, I punch 'Dementia and hallucinations' into Google.

***Hallucinations** are perceptions of objects or events involving the senses. They are real to the person experiencing them but cannot be verified by anyone else. Hallucinations experienced by people with Dementia can involve any of the senses – seeing, hearing, smelling, feeling or tasting – they are most often visual.*

A neuropsychologist I speak to months later – by which time the hallucinations have evicted most of Mum's reality so we seem to inhabit that alternate universe more than any real one – told me that hallucinations – and delusions – are not uncommon in Dementia, even if, she added, because she is aware this was the case for me, 'Carers are often shocked by them.'

In typical Alzheimer's disease, memory is usually affected first, then language. In the beginning, sufferers may struggle to find the right word. Then visual spatial ability is compromised, getting lost, which accounts for the wandering Dementia sufferers do. Then frontal lobe executive function is impaired, leaving it dented by disinhibition and delusions. The area of the brain that's affected last is the bit of the brain that's responsible for motor skills. I knew this was under attack months later when my mother's balance became so bad, she was not able to stand unaided. At about the same time, she developed such bad tremors in both arms she was unable to feed herself, or raise a cup safely to her lips. Hot tea became a hazard. There was something heart-breaking about not being able to share a fresh brew with her.

Delusions – believing things that aren't real – happen as a muddled combination of things: cognitive impairment and memory loss.

Say you put something down – a bunch of keys – and forget where you'd put them, you, I, would be able to rationalise where they may be. Retrace our steps. But in somebody with Dementia, the part of the brain that is responsible for rational thought isn't there anymore but – for a bit – the understanding that there must be an explanation for the fact of something 'missing' is. A rational thought then, when you can't find something you're looking for, could be 'I have been robbed, that's the only possible thing that can have happened.'

My mother – like Anthony Hopkins in *The Father* – began to fret about where her watch was, where 'all her money' had gone, who had stolen it. And then she began to accuse me of trying to poison her – persecutory delusions.

Why? Perhaps she perceived my insistence that she finish a drink as sinister; she could not comprehend the danger of dehydration, she did not feel thirsty, she could only feel the pressure of my wanting her to drain her glass. And what were all these pills for if she did not feel ill, why did she have to take them? Why did I – whoever I was – insist upon it? I *must* be trying to kill her, the only possible explanation.

But if it is skewed thinking that causes delusions, what caused my mother's visual hallucinations: what conjured those things into sight like a snake charmer luring a serpent from a basket? At first I wondered if it was some visual trick generated by her hemianopia, the condition that robbed her of right sided vision after her stroke. A blindness that left a space. A nothing. Possibly, but it was more likely the result of her Dementia-damaged brain as it began to trip up the senses she could once rely on, so that light, shadows, the movement of a curtain, conspired with her broken brain to endorse those tricks as fact.

The experts tell you to 'validate' a Dementia sufferer's belief; don't argue, just agree. Not just because it's pointless arguing with somebody who has Dementia but because, if you agree with them, they'll trust you. And – on a practical level – you need their trust to feed them, get them to drink, administer medication. On an emotional one, you need to be able to assuage some of the fear they feel. Distract where you can, say the experts. I try. 'How about a cup of tea, Mum?'

Until she cannot drink it anymore.

But on especially bad days – when she trusts nobody, when distraction has failed, when she sees men with guns rampaging across the lawn, when she hears voices and imagines people are living in the ceiling above her so that she puts a finger to her lips when I begin to speak, 'Shhh, or they'll hear you,' she whispers, gesturing upwards – on those days, Asina and I close the curtains to block out both the light and the nightmares and we turn up the music that has replaced the news channels on her radio.

And when even those things fail to rein in galloping monsters or weapon-wielding men or silence voices I cannot hear, an antipsychotic joins my mother's lengthy prescription and Asina and I score another line, creating a new column, in the notebook we keep to log the medicines Mum must take.

Before the antipsychotic was something to soothe night-time anxiety, manage the 'sundowning' which could keep her awake until sun-up, ignite her for 36-hour insomniac stretches at a time, in a strung-out state of high alert and distressing disconnection.

And before that, we added omeprazole to ease a digestion sluggish from a lack of activity and upset by an expanding list of medications.

It feels as if I'm trying to hobble my mother's body together as Alzheimer's tears her brain apart.

It feels like a race I am always losing. Some new hurdle presents, or presents differently, every week. Incontinence. Urinary first and then faecal.

If I notice any evidence of straining, I must titrate the doses of sickly-sweet stool-softening syrup up. Constipation in one so sedentary, whose appetite is so diminished now despite all the treats I nudge towards her, must be avoided at all costs.

I change my mother's diaper often, and still not nearly often enough. I smear the same nappy cream on the irritated skin of her buttocks as I did with my babies. This is harder with an adult. I cannot lie her on a changing mat and pick her ankles up with one hand to use the other to apply a protective barrier to breaking skin all the while blowing raspberries into her belly button. I must ask her to lie on her stomach on her bed so that I can peel her trousers down.

'Lie down how?' she wants to know.

There is pain in her back from sitting too long; pain in her knees from the creeping stiffness of inactivity; pain that she cannot describe.

I ask her, as I did my children when they were little and complained of some discomfort they did not have the language to articulate: 'Show me. Show me where it hurts.' I do not know if my mother's pain is real or imagined, if it is the perceived physicality of what is happening in her head.

I offer Mum painkillers anyway and instruct her on swallowing the two tablets I place on the flat of my hand.

She is forgetting even that: despite all the practice over all the years of all the hundreds of pills she's had to take, she cannot remember how to do this.

'Put them on the back of your tongue. No, no, not all together, one at a time. That's it – but right to the back of your tongue, right to the back,' I say and sometimes I must place a tablet there myself. And then I hold out a glass of juice: 'Take a big sip, Mum. That's right. Tip your head back. Swallow.'

Then, 'Gone? Has it gone?'

And – just like my children did – she opens her mouth wide and sticks out her tongue to show me.

I begin to use yogurt as a vehicle to get her medicines down – a spoonful of sugar, I think, as I crush the mirtazapine and lithium into full-fat saccharine strawberry-flavoured yogurt – is there any trace of real fruit in this? I worry – as I squash the pills into the pink.

As I mash, flecks of tablets fly to the floor and are lost. She will receive a reduced dose. But she is so reduced now, it will not matter.

We get a part of all six down that way.

And then Mum says, 'How will we get them out again?'

Out?

'How will we get what out, Ma?'

'Those pills.'

'Why would we need to do that?'

'You know: to sell them; we need to get them out to sell them.'

'We don't need to do that, Mum. They're yours. To keep.'

You will have conversations in Dementia that you'll never have in normal life about things you never imagined you'd have conversations about.

Sometimes – not often, but sometimes – she voices heart-breaking recognition that all is not well.

'I think I am going mad'

'Why, Ma?' I ask.

'Because I cannot think any thoughts. There is nothing in my head.'

'Shall we have a cup of tea?' I suggest, but cool, milky tea in a child's plastic sippy cup is not the same as a piping hot brew of builder's tea drunk from a bone-china mug you can cup your hands around.

Who tells you all this? Who tells you Dementia starts in the head and then hijacks the body so that one by one, as her mental faculties go, her physical abilities – to walk, to wipe herself, to register thirst or hunger, know where a pain is – do too?

There are drugs for all these things. All of them.

Except the one we need most.

* * *

Moving becomes especially hard. Mum leans backwards, as you might do if you were on water skis.

Postural inability: I learn the phrase a long time later; it happened very suddenly. One morning she could stand on her own. The next, her balance had gone: we had to pull her to her feet and the weight we bore in hands that tightly gripped hers told us she wouldn't stay upright on her own. I puzzle afterwards: did I imagine the severity and the suddenness of the change? 'You didn't,' an expert tells me: 'As Alzheimer's progresses, neurological decline can happen quite abruptly.'

She wobbles as she walks now, knees bent, feet tangling with every step so that I must keep reminding her, 'Keep your feet apart, Ma, feet apart, you'll be able to balance better then.'

'Oh yes,' she will say and she will stop and, with deliberation, plant her feet wide apart, so that for a moment, the briefest moment, she is steadier.

Some days are good. And some days are hard.

This evening, though, this evening is a good evening. Mum is calm. There is no evident pain. There is no fear.

'Shall we have a drink outside,' I suggest, 'and watch the sun going down?'

'Oh yes!' Her face lights up.

I wrap her up, I tuck a rug about her hips, across her stomach. I pull the zip of her fleece high. She is so thin now, the chill whips straight through her. I help her to the small patio outside her room.

I fetch a bowl and fill it with crisps. I nudge it in her direction, in the hope she may pluck the odd one out distractedly, from some long-buried snacking habit, and eat it.

I fill up her Coke. I call it beer. Like she used to drink. It sounds suitably grownup, inclusive. Celebratory. After all, this, this tiny achievement, outside, joining in, is worth drinking to.

I say 'Cheers' every few minutes – a prompt to raise her own glass, toast me and sip.

I point out the sun. It is sinking into the wild west saddle of the valley opposite us and north of the mountain whose bare shoulders begin to darken against the blush of sky.

Mum wants to know, where is the sun, and what is that big bright light (the sun) and are there more lights? And why are the clouds – are they clouds? – all yellow?

'That's the sun,' I say, 'it's lighting the clouds from beneath, as it sets.'

'Does this happen every day?' Mum asks.

Sunsets and sunrises. When Mum was well – hale, hearty, happy – when there was no sign of Depression's long shadow, my mother welcomed sunrises with tea and smiles. Eager for her day to begin, eager to get us up to celebrate this new-day energy with her, she would tap on doors armed with cups of tea for us too. When she was sick, she couldn't have cared less whether the sun ever rose again.

But sunsets. Sunsets were different; sunsets were always welcome – either for the simple fact of their splendour, or – when unwell – because they brought another difficult day to an end. Whatever her state of mind, there was something optimistic in the sun setting. (As opposed to sundowning, which Dementia has taught me bears nothing of the cheer of sunsets). On holiday, I noticed she selected postcards – counting off all the people she needed to send one to on her fingers – featuring sunsets, as if imparting some small omen of something hopeful to the recipient.

'Yup,' I say, 'It happens every day that the sun shines and the skies are clear.'

Every few minutes, between our raising glasses to one another, the same questions. Her gaze remains trained on the horizon which is distilled deep orange as whisky light spills and stains the last slip of sky.

And then it's gone and still she stays and remarks on the twinkling electric lights that sputter to life in her line of sight on the foothills and through forests. The cold begins to nip and I tell her it's time to go in.

I tell her we'll watch the sunset again tomorrow.

She will not remember today. She will enjoy it anew.

As if she'd never watched a sunset before.

Chapter 12: An Ebbing Tide

At ebb tide I wrote a line upon the sand, and gave it all my heart and all my soul. At flood tide I returned to read what I had inscribed and found my ignorance upon the shore.

– Kahlil Gibran

My husband asks me, 'What will you do if she dies?'

With time, the *if* morphs into *when*.

It's inevitable. Of course it is.

What will you do *when* she dies, as it becomes plain Mum is fading, as she eats less, moves less, sleeps more?

The end is coming and it is coming in a different guise than when it came for Dad: slowly, surely, not suddenly, unexpectedly.

Later, much later, in a conversation with a palliative care doctor, I will understand that avoiding the 'what to do if/when they die' conversation is not uncommon; even people whose parents are in their nineties resist it, she told me, 'As if they cannot accept the fact of a mother or father dying.' As if, in having that conversation, they are tempting fate, inviting the Grim Reaper over the threshold because he has heard his whispered name.

I ask my friend Marieke, who is familiar with the business of dying in remote Africa, what I need to do if-when Mum dies.

'There are graveyards in town,' she says, 'Is a Christian burial important?'

I have not considered this; I've never asked Mum, a mass-going Catholic most of her life, where – how – she wants to be laid to rest.

'There is also a Hindu crematorium,' Marieke continues, 'But it's an open pyre,' she warns.

I have witnessed this: an open-air cremation, a coffin balanced atop a pile of firewood, the steady lick of flames so that the sound of the fire and the hiss of traditional ghee used as fuel were all that filled my ears. That, and the insistent nag of the crows that watched from treetops. In India, the wealthy might instruct that the pyre be built of sandalwood for its perfume. Poor families must use whatever is at hand. Sometimes that means cow dung.

'It's a very spiritual spot, though,' Marieke says, 'Peaceful. And the trees are ancient and beautiful.'

When my father died, he was cremated. I still remember the jolt of shock when I saw his coffin, simultaneously for the first and last time, on a plinth in a modern crematorium. Was there any ceremony in the physical departure of that – as it slid behind a purple curtain and into a furnace? I could hear a distant roar, something many times larger and louder than when you turn on the gas ring of a hob. Later we were given a tinny urn of ashes. Were they even his, I wondered?

We buried them in one of the city's largest cemeteries, beside his brother, between his dead parents. In forty years, I have only visited the graveside once. I was warned, 'Don't go: there will be bandits and grave robbers,' but I went anyway and I stood and looked down at the marble headstone that bore my father's name and I felt nothing of him here. I did not linger.

I was too young to have the same conversation with my father: 'What shall we do with you when you die?' And I suspect he died too soon for my mother to have it either. I think if I had asked, Dad would have said that he would like his ashes to be spread somewhere with a view, somewhere where Africa spilled, careless and dusty, around him, some place where he could watch storms roll in and roll out and feel the rain above him and the sun beat down.

I know I need to have this conversation with Mum, but her comprehension is knotty and confused. I am uncertain how to do it without frightening her. Like many conversations, we have left it too late.

I fret about it for a bit, how to raise this sensitive subject with somebody who is cognitively challenged and wary of the prying of this sometimes-stranger.

Then I have an idea – I'll use the television as introductory medium. I scour Netflix and find something I think might work.

One afternoon Mum and I sit down to watch a programme about Varanasi, the sacred site where Hindus burn the bodies of their dead, where corpses swathed in saffron shrouds are laid on ghats on the bank of the Ganges and cremated so that afterwards, their ashes might float down the holy river and their souls be ushered to heaven.

I wonder if it will prompt the memory that India is where she was born. It does not.

But it does provide a helpful cue to the conversation I need to have about death.

'What a curious thing,' Mum says as she squints at the screen, 'People putting the dead in a river.' She is not perturbed by this, not repulsed or frightened, just puzzled.

Afterwards, sitting in the garden, I ask her: 'What shall

we do with you, Mum? When you shuffle off this mortal coil?'

I want to make it sound as if I am not asking a big question. But my once brilliant mother, her cognition dimmed, no longer gets innuendo.

'What?'

'When you die?' I elaborate, bluntly.

I can tell by her expression that this thought has not occurred to her: that we need to talk about when she dies. I have been struck at times that the more tenuous her grip on reality, the tighter her hold on life: she does not imagine she may be near the end of hers. She disputes her age often. 'I am sixty,' she insists. Whatever age she thinks she is, it's clear she does not think she is near the age she might die. Will she ever be? Or must we be in command of all our faculties to understand when life is worth living and when it is not? My grandmother wanted to die. At the end of her life, her thinking was still intact but her body was falling apart – blind, immobile, incontinent: 'I just want to go,' she said. And so I think: our instinct to survive, to *live*, is primal, it emanates from our animal brain. But our understanding of what it means to live *well* emerges from our intellectual self.

I soften my tone, 'We all have to go sometime, Mum.'

'I suppose so,' she agrees.

I describe my husband's communicated desire: 'He wants to be cremated,' I say, 'like the Hindus,' I prompt, 'but he doesn't want his ashes to be sent down a river, he wants them spread beneath a favourite tree in the garden, so he can hear the birds, enjoy the shade, admire the view.'

Why do we imagine this: that the dead could do all these things when they are ashes-to-ashes in an urn or scattered like seeds upon the ground, when there is nothing left of them but something softly composting, deep and moist?

Mum considers for a moment, 'Well, if you're still living here I suppose that would make sense, then you could sit with him and enjoy the view.'

Sit with him.

And so during our short conversation in the garden that afternoon, as sunlight filtered through the leaves of the tall trees my husband would like to lie beneath, I understand Mum thinks cremation makes more sense than a piling up of bodies, that she doesn't really care where what's left of her is buried, that she thinks my husband's idea, ashes in the garden, where she would be held in the deep embrace of an old tree's shadow, might be the perfect place to be laid to rest.

* * *

A dream.

My mother is beautiful. From a distance she looks young. Younger. I know that if I draw close, her age will show. So I watch her, from across a large room. She is dancing. Her partner, who is not my father, swings her around the floor and her expression is one of joy. I fear she may fall. Does he know how old she is, that man, I worry, how frail? I pitch myself forward in my seat ready to leap up if I need to. I keep watching. She dances on. And she is oblivious to me.

And then – in the way that dreams do – the direction and mood changes.

Now I arrive at an airport to find my mother there. She was meant to be gone. I know that her plane is many hours delayed, that she ought to have flown yesterday. She looks drawn, exhausted, sooty circles are smudged beneath her eyes. She stands when she sees me approach because she thinks she recognises me. I see uncertainty in her face and she falters. I know she is thinking, 'Do I know her?' I hasten forward, 'Mum,' I say, 'Mum, I'm so sorry.' She walks gingerly towards me, relieved that somebody she knows is here; at last, somebody she knows has turned up! *Where were we all*? As she moves, I see weariness. She is so tired her body almost tips forward, but I am there to catch her as she droops and in that vulnerability my temper flares. I shout at airport officials, 'She's been here all night. She's over eighty. Did nobody think to assist her?' They look right through me. They don't care.

My mother pats my arm, as if to soothe me. She is embarrassed by my histrionics.

'Shush, shush,' she says, 'It'll be okay, my plane will be here soon.'

And I wake and I think, even in my dreams my mother is leaving.

*

'You need to find out what to do when she goes,' my husband insists.

When she goes.

Perhaps if I never find out what to do when she dies, she never will?

We – my siblings and I (and Mum by default after our afternoon conversation on Varanasi) – have decided cremation is best.

I put that bit off – the where to burn her bit – until I grow so anxious about my mother's frailty I know I must know where I am going, where *we* are going, when it happens.

I text Eliza: 'Wondering about an outing to town next week. Market. To find crematorium. Will you come with me; I'll buy you lunch? X'

She says yes immediately. She says she wonders if anybody in the history of WhatsApp has received a message like that before. She sends me a kiss and a laughing emoji; she is already making this easier.

When we get to town, we can't find the Hindu pyre Marieke has told me about. And we don't know the Swahili word for crematorium. We only know how to ask where bodies are burned which sounds shocking when you say it out loud.

But Eliza worked for Reuters once, and in much more challenging places than this. She sleuths her way to the Hindu Temple.

'Let's start there, perhaps it's there,' she suggests.

We do. But it's not. The guards on the gate don't know what we're talking about. Eliza tries to describe dead bodies burning. They look more awe-struck than appalled at a beautiful 6ft blonde gesticulating wildly.

She flags down an Indian gentleman as he leaves the Temple and leans her tall, slender frame low to speak to him: 'Can you help?' she asks, 'We're looking for the crematorium.'

He can, he says with enthusiastic nodding. And he proceeds to direct us in quick-fire staccato. We think we've got it. We haven't. We peel off down road after road, asking a pedestrian here and a pedestrian there. Each gives us a different answer. We're going around in circles. We haven't got the right language yet. The right word. Google Translate is no help.

An African man wearing a bucket hat like the sort a trendy hipster might wear at Glastonbury is spreading rice and grain out to dry on sacks roadside. I stop to ask him.

His face lights up; he knows! 'Come, come,' he says, 'leave your car here and come.'

We are doubtful as we duck through a hedge and then down a narrow path on foot, 'Surely they don't expect you to carry your dead down this,' Eliza frowns.

We emerge in a clearing and find ourselves in a cemetery, weeds high as an elephant's eye. 'Here,' says the man in the bucket hat looking triumphant, 'Here are the dead.' We are standing, we realise from the configuration of the graves and the headstones, at the edge of the old Muslim cemetery.

'No, no,' and we explain again, as graphically as we dare, about the burning bodies. By then a small crowd has gathered, all intrigued by what we're doing, and they begin to chorus in unison: '*Makumbere! Makumbere ya Banyan*.'

Later I will find the literal translation for *Makumbere* in Kiswahili: 'shrine.' But in this context, our assembled helpers are referring to the Hindu crematorium we are looking for. And I will understand the reference to *Banyan* as soon as we find the right place minutes later: a small, gated glade at the end of a short road. There, in the centre of a shaded space, towering above an open pyre swept clean of any ash, is an enormous Banyan tree. It is majestic, its aerial roots a dense halo above the pyre. I grab Eliza's hand and hold it. This is where my mother will come when she dies, I know this.

I feel a surprising tranquillity soak through me. I don't feel fear and I don't feel revulsion. I feel sad but I feel calm.

That evening Eliza will send me a note to explain the significance of the Banyan

The Banyan tree is venerated in Hinduism because it lives for centuries and is considered God's shelter. Its large leaves

are often used in worship and rituals. The tree is a symbol of immortality; it represents the eternal cycle of death and rebirth; it protects spirits in the afterlife. Hindus believe the trees are inhabited by Gods and the spirits of deceased ancestors.

I write this now and think: Mum would have loved that tree, its spiritual story, our story. Our story that day would have made her laugh.

★ ★ ★

I can pinpoint the precise day my mother began to deteriorate. It began with a fall four months earlier. (Well, it began with Dementia – but you know what I mean). She fell early one morning before dawn.

Later I will understand why: she had developed the habit of taking her diaper off the moment she clambered out of bed. As if in disgusted disbelief at her failing body, she peels it down and abandons it on the floor. Or kicks it beneath something so it can't be found until later.

But she cannot make it to the loo without spilling the contents of her full night-time bladder on the bathroom floor. Pee on tiles is like black ice on a road; her feet skid out from beneath her and she lands with a crash, hitting the wall with her left shoulder on the way down.

Her wrist is already swelling by the time I get to her. Her shoulder looks foreshortened. There is pain. A lot of pain; a dislocation, I worry? A fractured wrist?

I sit her in a chair and remove her damp nightdress and replace it with something warm and dry as I urge her to sip hot sweet tea. She is being brave but shock is evident in her pale complexion.

Asina and I arrange her in the car. We pile cushions around her to protect her from jolts and I drive the two hours to the hospital.

I have avoided a trip to the doctor until now. Until now, Mum's body, her coming-undone head aside, has remained relatively well. Whatever small complaint arose in the past – indigestion, the flare of a rash, agitation, a sore on her skin – I could navigate with the help of medic friends. Sometimes I sent descriptions of ailments or photographs via WhatsApp to my local pharmacist. But this is too big to deal with virtually.

Bruises are beginning to bloom by the time Mum is wheeled into the emergency room. Their darkness reflects in the shadows that skitter across the medics' faces: Did she get these in the fall?

'Yes.' I say. 'Yes, she did.'

The oximeter plugged onto a finger indicates low oxygen levels.

'We need to do a chest X-ray,' they say.

'What about her shoulder?' I insist, 'Her wrist?' I say. Her wrist has lost its slender proportions. It's ballooning and blackening.

'We'll get to those: we are worried about pneumonia.'

'*Pneumonia*?!'

I am startled: 'Wouldn't there have been coughing? A fever? Breathlessness?'

They ignore my question and ask one of their own: 'Has she ever smoked?'

'Never,' I say.

'Lived with a smoker?'

Does my father count? A sixty-smokes a day man until he was killed almost forty years ago.

'No,' I say: It's easier to explain that way: 'No.'

'Is she on any meds?'

'Yes. Lots.' And I list them: anti-anxiety tablets, antidepressants, blood thinners, lithium…

'Lithium?'

'Yes, lithium.'

My mother keeps tugging the nasal cannula out of her nose: 'It's making my nose run, take it out,' she whines

'Your nose isn't running, Mum,' I reassure her.

'It's the humidity,' the nurse explains, 'We mix the oxygen with water otherwise it would be too dry and would make your nasal passages uncomfortable.'

Too much information. Mum looks blank but acquiesces: 'Okay.'

Five minutes later, she's tugging at it again: 'Take it out, take it out, it's making my nose run.'

I have explained in a quiet aside to the attending physicians, 'She has Dementia.'

Carer-speak for: 'Direct all questions to me – even the ones about her name and where she lives.' In fact, especially those. And be sensitive – for God's sake, be sensitive.

My mother has only heard the word once in context to her condition: *that means I am demented.*

A team crowds around her. 'So,' they say loudly, and over Mum's head: 'She has Dementia.'

My mother might have lost her memories, but she hasn't lost her hearing. Her eyes widen in horror. I feel my hackles rise. I frown a warning at the assembled medics. I indicate the affirmative with a tiny, curt nod and hope Mum does not see.

We need to do an ECG, the doctors insist and bustle into Mum's cubicle wheeling an electrocardiogram machine. Then they draw the curtains around her bed.

I hear her from behind pale blue drapes explaining the anatomical defect she was born with:

'My breast on that side never grew properly.'

Silence. Which prompts her to explain:

'I was born like that.'

She remembers this congenital shortcoming. A left clavicle that does not match the right; one breast deflated, one still round and plump.

'My horrid little boob,' she has said to me.

Her spine now twists and curves, contorted by her shrunken side.

X-Rays of her shoulder, her arm, her wrist are all normal: there are no fractures. Perhaps a sprain, the doctors say. That, and their expressions grow dark, 'That and the bruising.'

When her chest X-ray comes back, they tell me: 'Yes: pneumonia: white spots all over her lungs.'

I must look doubtful – at this incidental finding, that it could be so serious – for they invite me over to their screens to look.

'See? This is what a healthy lung should look like,' they point. I noticed they have punched 'healthy lung' into Google images. And I think wryly, so it's not just me.

'Look: this is your mother's: see all those white spots. Pneumonia!'

There is the faintest dappling on my mother's image, as if somebody had spread a cobweb across it. More than that, though, much more than the chalky dusting across the darkness, I notice how crumpled my mother's left lung looks, as if it's being crowded out by a collapsing skeleton. As if one birthday balloon was still buoyantly blown up and the other sagging miserably under some invisible weight. Deflated since birth.

'I see,' I say. I don't.

'We need to admit her.'

'Why?' I ask.

'Because she has pneumonia,' and, in case I don't know what pneumonia is, 'An infection in her lungs.'

'Yes but there were no clinical signs of this,' I insist. 'I brought her in because she fell; I was worried about her shoulder, her wrist, not her breathing. She was fine yesterday: up, about, walking, eating.'

Mum, who might have enjoyed the first flurry of attention, who might briefly have been interested in the machines and bleeps to begin with, is growing agitated. She keeps pulling the oximeter off her finger so that the monitor above her bed screams and the pulsing green line flatlines. She tugs the nasal cannula from her nose, again and again, tying its tubes in knots about her throat. She squirms away from the blood pressure cuff, the doctor wriggles it on anyway and Mum begins to wail, 'Ow, ow, ow' as it inflates and tightens around her upper arm.

'When is lunch?' she wants to know, 'Have I even had my breakfast? And where is my daughter?

'WHERE IS MY DAUGHTER?' she demands again, loudly: 'I WANT MY DAUGHTER.'

'I'm here, Mum,' I say, 'I'm here,' and I pop my head through her curtain to reassure her, 'I'm just here.'

She looks at me: 'Thank God, I thought you'd gone.'

'I don't think it'd be wise or kind to admit her,' I tell the medical team. Then, in a whisper at a distance from Mum's bed, 'Her Dementia is advanced, this will confuse her, distress her, cause even more regression.'

'I want to go home,' Mum wails, from behind her curtain: 'Please can we go home?'

'Of course, Mum,' as I move to shush and try to placate and offer her another biscuit and a sip of juice, as you might a fractious toddler.

'We could put her in a VIP room.'

A VIP room. I almost laugh: what good will that do, sleeping in a strange room, nights broken by the entry and exit of unfamiliar faces, the shriek of sirens, a room too hot, too bright, too loud? What of that will be eased by the prestige of the ward?

'Can we show you a menu of rooms available,' they offer, 'with prices?'

This is not about cost. I'd pay anything to mend my mother's broken brain.

'No. No I don't think so: she's not staying.'

They grow alarmed and persuasive and when that does not work, they produce a disclaimer form and point to the place where they need my signature: I must sign where it says, 'The risks of refusing admission have been explained to me.' They include death.

I say: 'So this is absolving you of responsibility, if something happens?'

'Yes,' they say, 'if something happens...'

They don't say: 'You are taking her home to die.' They don't need to.

But here, if I leave her here, will they put her chair out in the sun in the morning so she can hear the birds and watch the view? No, they will not. There are no birds. There is no view. Will they cater to a failing appetite? Tempting it with things I know she likes but they will not: egg sandwiches with too much salt; dark chocolate; strawberry yogurt. A beer at sundown? I don't think so. Is there a cat to sleep on her bed? A dog to sit by her chair to chuck scraps at and talk nonsense to? No. There are none of these few things that ground her, make her feel safe, cherished.

I am not taking her home to die. I am taking her home to *live.*

★

She sits in the back of the car, like a little bird with a broken wing, safe in her nest of pillows. She gazes out of the window all the way home. She is delighted when we get there. Today she remembers what home means. It means her chair, her telly, her bedroom and the dog she has grown so fond of. She tells me over and over how happy she is to be here and not 'in prison'.

She forgets about her fall within hours. Instead she puzzles that she cannot move her left arm. She is childlike in her pride of the bruising which runs from her shoulder to her elbow.

She shows it to everybody she talks to on Skype: 'See my arm?' she asks, twisting in her chair, clumsily trying to position herself so whomever she's talking to has a view of it: 'Have you seen the funny colour my skin has gone?'

We were lucky Mum didn't break anything. Her fall is not the end. But it is the beginning of the end. Her movement is hampered with only one working arm and, even when her bruised arm regains some movement, it is weak and twitches. Being able to only bear weight on one arm means getting in and out of chairs and up and down from the loo is impossible. She needs more help.

And because of that, she grows more helpless.

★ ★ ★

It is Mum's birthday. She's 82. Except I have lied. About the date.

'Happy Birthday, Mum,' I say.

'Is it my birthday? '

'It is,' I say, 'Do you know what the date is?'

'Of course,' she says, 'If it's my birthday, it must be the 9th of June, I'd never forget *that*.'

But it's not the 9th. It's the 11th. On the 9th I was at the memorial service of an old friend of mine, of Mum's. You do your best. You split your time. You lie about dates when it doesn't matter.

'Whose memorial?' Mum had asked when I told her I was going.

She remembers the name, she says. Like she sometimes remembers mine. Or – more rarely – Dad's. She recalls the names of real people she once knew, but she can't tell me the names of the imaginary people she sees every day; her paranoia is growing worse, her hallucinations more vivid and compelling.

'Have I told you the secret I told her?' Mum whispers, gesturing somebody who isn't there.

'What secret? Who?'

'Her. *Her*! THAT secret,' the careless sweeping of a hand that she makes every time I don't understand.

'*My* secret,' delivered in a hush, a clandestine hiss.

'I'll ask her later,' I say, 'I'll ask her later to tell me the secret you told her.' Whoever she is.

'NO! NO! Don't. Don't mention it. Please don't.'

Secrets and suspicion, they lend the ugly weight of nothingness to nothing. Layer it all up and lend more invisible weight to this vanishing illness. How can something of no substance feel like the heaviest thing in the world?

Before you know it, you are casting bricks from some intangible matter – helium or hydrogen or pixie dust, something fine as ash and light as a feather.

This, this growing madness, is shocking.

'Shhhh,' hisses Mum, eyes round, finger to lips, 'Or they might hear us.'

'They?'

'In the roof,' she says, indicating upward with a subtle inclination of her head.

There are interviews, up there, apparently, being conducted by people she can hear and I cannot. One. Two. Three. There are questions. Four. Five. Six.

There are no answers.

She is trying to make sense of the cat's cradle cast of Alzheimer's in her mind. And as I listen to her, I think of Russell Crowe as John Nash and a garden shed papered with press cuttings and webbed with string as schizophrenia crazy-paved his thoughts.

Later she will tell me, still seized by invisible terror, 'I cried and I cried'

'Why Mum, what made you cry?'

'Because I wish I were not so unbrave.'

Unbrave? My mother who wrestled black dogs, navigated life as a young widow after my father's shocking death, learned to read again because she could not imagine a life without words, hard won words which this horrid disease is stealing from her anyway?

What has happened to my brave mother's Beautiful Mind?

★

That day, though, the birthday that wasn't her birthday was a peaceful day, her demons leave her alone and I make a birthday cake. Lemon. I hope the tart sweetness will pinch her tastebuds awake. Chocolate is too risky; she'll toss it to the floor when she thinks we are not looking, where the Labrador will snaffle it up and then have an allergic reaction (and I can do without the drama). So lemon it is. I bake a sponge to her recipe.

Six ounces of everything, she used to say: 'Six of butter, sugar, flour and three eggs, or eight of everything to four eggs. Easy multiples. It's as simple as that,' she smiled.

It was. Once.

And for the icing, to cinch the two halves together in a bitter-sweet kiss, I make lime curd using the double boiler Mum gave me decades ago and, as I stir, I remember how she stood over me as a child, helping me make curd for the Home Economics stand at the local agricultural show, how she behaved as if I'd won an Oscar when my jar of preserve was Highly Commended.

I light the candle I have plonked on the top which I've dredged with icing sugar. We sing happy birthday to her. She looks perplexed. She smiles. She says thank you.

She opens the present we gift her: a scarf she already owns and loves but does not remember is hers.

I don't know if she nibbles a second tiny slice of cake because she likes whatever she tastes, or because she doesn't want to hurt my feelings.

We sit on the patio, late afternoon sun is sieved through the fat foliage of the tree above us – a tree she has admired often for its dense branches and the umbrella of shade it gives. Sometimes she would look for birds up there, craning her neck from where she sat beneath it. When she was first here, she would try to mimic their calls, asking me what I thought they were saying.

It's a warm evening but I must cover Mum up in blankets and a thick fleece. I wrap the new-old scarf around her neck.

'How lovely and soft this is,' she says.

I toast her with a glass of wine. She reciprocates with her Coca-Cola.

But the afternoon is brief.

'I think I'd like to go in now,' she says and so I help her rise from her wheelchair and walk her up the shallow ramp into her room.

I watch a short video my husband took that day now and I am horrified at how enfeebled Mum had grown, how thrown her balance, how buckled her knees, how she barely lifted her Dementia-friendly-slippered feet to take the smallest, shuffling steps as I, walking backwards, dragged her forward, straining to keep her upright.

What do I do with all the memories? That sweet memory of her last birthday, a sunny afternoon? What do I do with all the memories she cannot – could not – hold, could not keep in her leaky-bucket brain? How will I preserve them?

If only I could bottle them as I did my curd, a waxed lid to protect them from decay, and a prize for my efforts.

*

A week later and I can almost feel death's cold breath on my neck. Will it come as she sleeps? Is the pain she describes in her chest a pulled muscle (from the little effort she exerts), a bruise, where I have grabbed her in panic as I lower her to the loo and her legs give way? Or as I manoeuvre her into the shower, navigating a slippery-when-wet floor?

Or is it something more sinister? Her heart? Her lungs?

I place my hand on my own heart and feel its steady, sturdy rhythm against my palm.

She is breathless, 'I've just had a run, you see,' she tells me.

'Should I take her to hospital?,' I ask my husband, my brother, my sister, Mum's sister who was a nurse for many years. And I know as I ask, it is mostly fear that prompts my question: do I have the courage to sit with my mother to the end? My aunt kindly, firmly reminds me of the Hippocratic oath.

Thou shalt not kill; but needst not strive, ***officiously****, to keep alive.* 'Officiously,' she repeats.

Officiously.

I look the word up now.

Intrusively enthusiastic.

And I will remember in my asking that Mum and I had a conversation about this, at least, even if we didn't have a conversation about 'What to do with you when you die?'

'If I ever have an illness that cannot be cured, I don't want any heroics,' Mum had said, 'No invasive, painful treatments to no end.'

I recall being shocked at the time, at her calm acceptance of what she considered fate.

But if I was shocked then I am grateful now, for that long-ago instruction: I could not subject my mother to the fear of a strange hospital again, the machines, the tubes, the discomfort, the confusion of not understanding who's who or where she is or why.

I could not do that to her. For what? To delay her dying by a day? Two? To fill her last hours with terror and loneliness?

No, I have to be brave. I must watch this slow going. I must stay calm so Mum does too. Later, a long time later, a doctor will say to me, 'There are better ways to die than Dementia,' and I will wonder, did I at least help her to a better death?

I offer her two paracetamols for the ache she describes, which she tells me she got when she fell while getting onto the ship.

'Will the journey be a long one?' she wants to know.

'I don't know. I don't think so,' I say.

Even in her dying she is showing me courage.

Two days later she says she wants to die.

★

And two days after that, a Monday morning near the end of June when I go to wake her, I find her bed is unruffled, as if she has lain deathly-still all night. I urge her up and peel the covers back. She looks, then, naked of her duvet, like a corpse might look entombed in a coffin, curled and skeletal, her hands clawed, her cheeks sunken.

She says she is very tired, 'I should like to stay in bed today.'

Exhaustion is stealing her voice so that the sound of it is small and soft and I must bend close to hear her.

'That's okay, Mum, you do that. You have a rest,' and I tuck her up again.

She smiles gratefully at me and closes her eyes.

Later, propped up, I will hold a slice of bread to her mouth and urge her to take a bite.

'Just a little bite; it's got honey on it, Ma, you love honey.'

In force-feeding her, I am sustaining her. How do you know what's right to do? When should I stop this? This is all that keeps her alive now, my determination to keep pushing food and fluids into her.

I give up with the bread and pick up her juice and hold it

to her lips. She takes a tiny sip, then, 'That's enough now,' she says, turning her face away.

On Tuesday she calls me by her beloved sister's name. She keeps calling me by that name. Because she knows me? Because she doesn't? Because she can trust me. She asks me to go away. She asks me to stay. She thanks me. Over and over and over. Thank you, thank you. A sip of juice here. A wet flannel pressed to lips there.

Everything about sitting by and watching, waiting, is counter to my nature: I want to force fluid into her, I want to add oxygen and push her full of the fuel to keep going. I want to *fix* her.

But I cannot fix her brain.

She folds her hands together. 'I want to say my prayers now. Good night,' she says. It's not even noon. She keeps saying it, her hands this-is-the-church-this-is-the-steeple clasped together. I dig in drawers for her rosary. I can't find it and can't imagine where it's gone and I feel a great anger at myself for being so unprepared.

★

The days blur now. I don't remember much of what happened when or next or how. Mum is still and quiet. I sit by her bed.

Sometimes I lay my head on it and doze for a while. Once – once not long ago – she'd have reached a hand across to comb her fingers through my hair.

I spend the night like that. Two. I hear nightjars, a beetle and Mum's breath, the rise and fall, as if in dream or on the move.

In the small, lonely hours of the second last night, I scour the internet for tips on how to face what is coming. I stumble across a Ted Talk by palliative care doctor Kathryn Mannix.

I watch it with tears streaming down my face and my earpods in so that Mum can't hear. And then I understand what to expect: what Mum might look like as she goes, what she may sound like. What the 'death rattle' means. I know not to be alarmed by it. I am aware I am approaching even this forensically, this urgent habit of questioning shaped by my mother, because in asking, I will be better prepared.

I tap a message to Mannix on Instagram into my phone.

I read your book ages ago but at the time it was somewhat academic; I had never witnessed a death. Now I find myself at my dying mother's bedside, late-stage AD. Feeling fearful of what was to come, I found you again online, a YouTube video, Dying for Beginners. I wanted to tell you how calming and reassuring I have found your words. Thank you for bringing death back into everyday conversation and making me feel stronger when I needed to be.

She responds within hours – and in time: *I'm so sorry you're in this poignant situation. I hope your mother is calm and comfortable. Remember unconscious people still hear so your familiar voice will be a gift to her. You can do this.*

So I keep talking to Mum. I play music. My children, my siblings, send voice notes for me to play so that virtual conversations hum all night. I massage Mum's hands and her feet and I notice the mottling of her skin where blood is pooling and stagnating, as her heart slows and her circulation stalls. I brush her hair. I had cut and washed it only days before and it feels thick and glossy beneath the bristles.

'Let's wash your hair,' I had said, one slow afternoon when she had seemed especially unhappy.

I could not remember the last time we'd washed it. I felt ashamed of that. But Mum's lack of mobility, her curled spine, who would notice if it wasn't clean anyway…

But but but.

It had grown too long. She looked wilder and madder as a result.

I set up an arrangement at her basin, I fashioned a tall seat out of her walker so that she could sit as I shampooed, I draped towels over her lap and shoulders to keep her dry because by then she was unable to bend her head low enough to the sink. Water went everywhere. She didn't mind. She clutched the towel about her shoulders, covering her nose with it. I massaged her scalp and soon her hair was thick with foam. Rinsed, I rubbed it dry.

'Shall we cut it, Mum?'

She did not ask whether I had any experience of cutting hair. Maybe she didn't care. Maybe she trusted me enough to try.

And so, with a pair of blunt paper scissors so that I sliced more than snipped, I feigned proficiency, made her laugh with stories of how I used to cut my children's hair, how it looked as if I'd demarcated the cutting line with a pudding basin, how none of them would let me near them now. More hair than I imagined came off. Rained to the floor like ash and puddled there. Later I held up a mirror to show her.

'Gosh,' she said with a smile, 'It really did need a cut.'

Now it is I who combs my fingers through her still shampoo-perfumed hair, I stroke the dome of the head I cupped days ago as I rinsed suds from silvering tresses.

*

How long will this take? Too long and not long enough? I want to spirit her to wellness. I want Asina to sing-song her way into Mum's room and bossily instruct, in better-by-now English, 'Time for go walking, Lala.' I want her to help me hoist Mum to her feet and lead her into the garden. I want to drink a beer with Mum as the sun goes down. I want to say all the things I did not say because what was the point, she'd forget anyway. I want to say them over and over and over.

I am full of sadness and full of guilt. All the things I could have done and did not do. Did I know this guilt would gnaw? Did I? Did I do enough? I will always think I didn't, as I excused myself with work and marriage and things I had to do. This is the curse of caring, I learn later: you do what you can and afterwards you are consumed by remorse that what you could do wasn't enough.

Asina puts head around the door to check where we are in this slow, sad journey. I motion her towards me. She draws a chair to Mum's bedside and we sit together, quietly. This collaboration which has sung with communication as we tried over months to fathom what now, what next, is silenced: There are no words.

There is a flicker of a pulse at Mum's wrist, a tap-tap that I watch and am hypnotised by. A metronome that slows and jerks. Was it always like this? Is there a small vascular deformity here or is it like this because she is going? I have never thought to examine my mother's pulse before. It is like a tiny lighthouse caught beneath the skin.

Hours later and I try to find it again. But its beat is thready, thinner. I must try hard to feel for it now, my fingers fumbling to find it as her fingers grow pale and cold. It is as if something has turned down a fire inside her.

She grows colder. Asina wraps her up tight in her duvet, tucks her old-new scarf uselessly around her neck, we will not stem this chill.

Why is she crying, Asina wants to know, worried, as Mum's eyes, half-mast, brim and spill with tears.

I tell her what I have only understood in recent hours and only then because I sought Dr Mannix out in the ether: 'She isn't, Asina, she just isn't blinking anymore.'

I learned that face muscles relax completely close to death. And with that relaxation, a person can no longer close their eyes, their tear ducts stop working, the water that wells there leaks. Mum sheds tears but she isn't weeping. Her mouth falls open, as if in the deepest sleep.

Asina is satisfied for a moment.

And the noise, she frets, at every deep rattling breath Mum struggles to take, 'Why is she making that noise? Is she in pain?'

'No Asina' and I tell her what Mannix also taught me the night before: that Mum could no longer feel fluid collecting in her throat, was so relaxed she no longer had the urge to cough to clear it. It was simply gathering there, shallow breaths bubbling through it.

We sit there then, in the gathering gloom. Asina holds Mum's hands, I sit on Mum's bed behind her so that I can envelop her in a hug.

She does not go until the chill has reached her shoulders. I hold her tight. I kiss her. I tell her she can let go, that her job is done.

And then there it is: her last breath.

And she is gone.

Just like that: She is gone.

The hardest thing. Letting her go and willing her to stay.

She goes as the sun sinks. If she could have seen it – that last vivid, tangerine ripe sunset – she'd have loved it.

*

'Do not cry,' Asina admonishes as she witnesses me begin to weep, 'There is work to be done, you can cry later.'

She has never seen a person die either but 'my mother has,' she confides now, 'She has told me what to do. We need to wash Lala before she dries out.'

We bathe and change Mum while she is still soft and yielding before the stiffness of death makes it impossible. Tenderly, Asina taking charge, we lay her out on the floor. We peel off a nightgown damp with her last perspiration. We sponge her with warm – for Asina insists it must be and waits until the hot tap steams – soapy water. We pat her shrunken body dry with a fresh towel. Asina collects the talc Mum used after every shower and liberally douses her body with it. We dress her in a favourite kanzu of vibrant orange and sky blue. I brush her blow-away clean hair. We lift her, suddenly surprisingly heavy in her deadweight, and lay her on fresh sheets. For months afterwards I will reflect on this intimacy shared between Asina and I in Mum's last hours. I will be reminded of a similar intimacy between a birthing mother and a midwife and I will wonder at the women who helped my mother bring me into the world as Asina and I accompanied her out of it.

I kiss her a last time. I push her bedroom window wide open to the cool night and the insistent shriek of bush babies.

*

She was cremated the next day at the Hindu crematorium.

My champions in this – Ant, Asina in her best dress, Eliza and Marieke – stood beside me.

My siblings and I thought it was a fitting end, the neat closing of a circle, Indian birth, Indian death: *the eternal circle.*

I swear I could hear my maternal grandmother's approving murmurs; perhaps her spirit was wound in the branches of the Banyan tree above Mum. The pyre was lit to the chanting of Hindu prayer – Gran would have loved that too.

⋆ ⋆ ⋆

In the weeks before Mum died, I watched her turn the pages of her wedding album. 'I expect that's my husband,' she had said of the man whose hand she held in the pictures.

But on the anniversary of Dad's death – six days before her own – Mum will keep asking, 'Is your father coming? When is he coming?'

How come she knows he is my father now?

Did she know she was leaving?

In the nights before she died, she began putting a framed photo of Dad under her pillow. I laid the same photo on her chest as she was lowered onto the pyre. I sent them off together.

I will collect her ashes later. I put them in a wooden urn, carved as a globe. It does not close evenly where it is meant to screw shut around its equatorial girth so that none of the countries line up; nothing is where it's meant to be, and that seems appropriate.

I will – in time – find precisely the right tree in precisely the right spot.

I will sit with her and we will enjoy the view together. Perhaps I will drink a cold beer for us both.

⋆

Later, I will look in the fridge and see all the things I bought for Mum, to try to tempt her appetite: yogurt, cheese,

KitKats, thick, sweet mango juice, a lot of Coca-Cola. I will smell the pumpkin soup we made just days before she died, dense with the scent of cinnamon, and I will wonder, 'Will the spicy perfume of it haunt me forever, will an old memory of its scent be usurped by this new one?' What happens to memories of things as they change – as the plump smell of sweet happiness is thinned by Dementia?

It is the gut-punches afterwards that get me.

The full packet of Weetabix, the unopened tubs of vanilla ice cream, the digestive biscuits – these things were her staples at the end. I never eat them.

A small ball of cotton wool when I open a box of ear drops. I administered them to her for a few days when she complained of soreness. I had tucked the cotton wool into the box afterwards so that I could stuff it into her ear to keep the oily drops from dribbling down her jaw. 'Next time,' I had said, 'We'll use this bit of cotton wool next time.'

But next time never came.

It is these small things that hit hardest in grief.

The smell of the talc which she used to dust herself with after a shower. I watched it snowstorm across her stomach, which got more shrunken with every week. A wizened child shape beneath an old lady's skin.

A roll of micropore tape I must rip a couple of inches from three weeks after she dies when I cut my thumb slicing aubergines. Its end is ragged and difficult to unpick. I tore it off in haste, to tape Mum's eyes shut after she died. I wanted her to appear asleep, not dead-eyed and staring.

The Tupperware I bought to keep her biscuits fresh, still almost full. One is broken in half. Did I snap it in two and try to tempt her with the other half? At the end of her life, even those were tipped to the floor for Jip, or stashed in pockets for me to find later. Soft and crumbling. Like her.

For weeks after she goes, I cannot go into her room. I cannot even look at it; I cannot lift my head to her windows as I go past them.

For weeks, I keep my head down, a palm raised as a blinker whenever I approach the house after a walk because the view of her window will be the first thing I see as I round a final bend. A window that told me, when she was still here, how the day had begun. On dawn walks, when I rounded that bend, I would find curtains open on good days and I might see the shape of her beyond and know that she was up and making tea. But with time, as her brain laid waste to her body and she was unable to rise unaided, those curtains stayed drawn; she relied on us to let the light in.

It was from that same window that I could point out a full fat moon. I would switch off all the lights behind us so that we were plunged into the dark and I'd open the curtains she'd closed earlier and I'd point.

'There Mum, do you see it? The moon.'

It took her time to locate it, which puzzled me: it was so round, so plump, the pale face of it tilted down as if it too was urging her: 'Look! I'm up here. See!'

'Look up, Mum,' I'd say, and sometimes I might put a finger beneath her chin to lift her view and then:

'Oh yes. Oh gosh!' And we'd watch it together for a while.

On many evenings she watched the sunset from the other side of the same room, the last light of day in those twilight weeks. I opened the curtains wide – the ones I'd closed against invisible soldiers wielding guns in the garden earlier – and I'd let the night settle around us. And Mum would drink in that whisky-spill of dusk, see it distil in glass panes and puzzle at where the sun was going.

But afterwards? Afterwards I cannot look at her windows. I cannot look at them in daylight where I will not see her drawing curtains wide. I cannot watch them after dark for there are no lights burning there, lights which I would sometimes be frustrated to see blazing in the middle of the night.

Then one day I try, six weeks after she goes, I tell myself to get over myself: lift your head and look. Not at the moon like I'd told Mum to do. But at those empty windows. I make myself. I take a deep breath in as if I were diving into water, and I force myself to look, but the sting is too much.

I lower my head and feel tears spill.

When Dad died there was no looking into the places where he had been; we upped and left and that was that.

I cannot decide if this is better, if this makes growing accustomed to empty spaces easier, this sitting, literally, so close to where she was. Forcing myself to stare into my grief. Into windows. I knew she was dying so this sadness is not the shocking slap of Dad's death which left me numb. There is no numbness here, just a deep, deep ache. And every time I look up, every time I see those curtained windows, a room shuttered up, folded away, cold and wanting, it's a thumb pressing into a bruise.

And yet, curiously, despite the visceral experience of her death – the sitting with her until the very end, the way her face changed in dying, the waxy pallor that replaced the pink of her complexion, the iciness of that creeping chill as the flame of life was extinguished – despite witnessing all that, there were no nightmares afterwards. Six months later and my dreams of Mum, if I have them at all, are gentle ones.

I dream Mum and I are at a party together. By the sea. The occasion is in celebration of her. But I cannot be certain why; maybe in my dream it is the last party we will hold for her. My mother sits at the other end of a long table from me. I keep an anxious eye on her. I can hear the music of my childhood, Bert Kaempfert's 'That Happy Feeling'. In another life, in real life, I had watched the LP being slid from its sleeve and wiped on my mother's own. Then, with edges gripped between palms so it wasn't smudged or scratched, the record was placed gently on the turntable, the needle lowered and the orchestra struck up. I saw my father take one of Mum's hands in his, wrap an arm around her waist and sweep her across a room as he led her in a dance. And even at five I knew I was witnessing something that did not include me, something intimate. In my dream, I suddenly notice mum is no longer at the end of the table. She's vanished. I rise, worried, to find her. But there she is, leaning against a wall, watching the slip of the day, the last lights linger. It is I who takes her hand now, to guide her slowly down steps to her room. She is leaving in the morning. I promise her I will get up early to help her pack. I notice she is wearing yellow heels. She never wore yellow heels.

She turns to say goodnight, 'Thank you, I have had such a wonderful time.'

The next morning, I search for Kaempfert's compositions on Spotify. The app offers me the soundtrack to *Still Alice*.

Three months after Mum died, we held a memorial for her in Northamptonshire, not far from where she lived for twenty-five years. We organise a Catholic mass to honour her faith, one she encouraged us towards with a gentle take-it-or-leave-it nudge. She did her best while at the same time trying not to laugh at our resistance. As young children, and in the absence of an English-language option, she felt compelled to take us to a long Swahili service in a hot church on Sundays. We observed – watchful through the tedium of a sermon we could not understand – that the church doors were locked soon after the priest took to the pulpit: latecomers were not tolerated. And so began a crusade of last-minute lost shoes and urgent trips to the loo just as Mum herded us all into the car.

'Come on, kids, we're going to be late' (which was, of course, the point).

Successfully deterred, we'd arrive to find the doors shut tight. Mum would sigh, roll her eyes at us and instruct a quick prayer in the car. Piously – jubilantly – we'd put our palms together and whisper fervent thanks.

Mum's memorial mass is a small and intimate affair. And it is not the music – John Barry's 'Flying Over Africa' – nor the faces of family members, nor even my brother's moving eulogy when he remembered our childish attempts to thwart Mum's efforts to get us to church on time ('Thank you, Father Paul, for opening the doors of the church for us today,' he smiled), which make my tears flow. No, those come later, as I drive through the once familiar Northamptonshire countryside, which spills wide and pale in late summer sunshine and which I have not returned to for more than a decade. I had forgotten the size of those fields, so big that one near Mum's long-ago village was nicknamed Little America. I cry when I see signs for the A509.

'Take that exit off the M1,' Mum told me the first time I drove home from London, 'The 509's the best route.'

Grief finds us in funny places. We don't know what reminders people will leave until they are gone: road signs, supermarkets. It is the simplest things that winkle out some deep part of you that is buried, some long ago memory of sweet ordinariness: my mother asking my children what they wanted to do when we visited her in England: 'Go to Tesco,' they chorused.

And so she took them, all three, vibrating with excitement, and she put one in a trolley and the other two held either side of it. She took her time trawling aisles and filling her cart with things she'd never buy normally. Petit Filous, Creme Caramel (which she taught them how to eat – tipping the container onto a saucer so that the burned sugary sweetness ran down the sides of a small custard mound), chocolate mousse in little pots, which she encouraged them to fill to the brim with cream, then dig a spoon in so that they could create a well for a little more.

I stood in the same supermarket the week of Mum's memorial and wept as I gazed at pots of yogurt in the chilled section of the store.

My youngest daughter remembers some of this in her tribute to her grandmother that day in a pub garden where we gather under skies which are too blue and a sun so Africa-hot we must all shed jackets and come home with sunburned noses. She remembers that her grandmother's generosity with anything chocolate was in stark contrast to her mother's spartan sharing of a single Mars Bar among the five of us. That made us all laugh.

I read the last pages of Octavia Bright's *This Ragged Grace* through tears. Her father's experience of Alzheimer's was both different from Mum's and the same. In the end, they are all the same: the slow going: 'It's easier to understand the kind of dying that's contained and immediate. For most, the ongoingness of a drawn-out death is a horror too far,' Bright wrote.

This is the great sadness of caring for somebody you love with Dementia. Its slow, cold creep means that years are spent wading through its watery fallout, groping and uncertain, always feeling out of your depth. And as this illness drowns out everything about this person you love, it changes them, so you begin to lose sight of them; it diminishes them so they become a dot on your horizon.

A high tide, a rising wave that alters the shape of the shore and flattens sandcastles.

But if you reach back, if you reach back to before all this and look, they're still here, always here, in surprising, everyday spaces.

Months after mum dies and I keep finding her: a hairbrush on a bathroom shelf, strung with silver mined from her scalp, that last long evening as I brushed her hair. An almost empty tube of moisturiser. I slice it open with a pair of scissors. I scrape it clean and massage the cream into my skin as I stand in front of a mirror. I see tears well. Mum taught me this trick. Here she is now, again, a lifetime after I first watched her do this with a tube of Elizabeth Arden. I stumble upon an old exercise book. The cover bears the words, 'Christmas Card List' in Mum's handwriting. The stroke of her pen is achingly familiar. I have seen that neat slant on a thousand letters, an envelope at boarding school that bore my name in her signature script brought something of deep reassurance. Her DNA doesn't just ribbon mine; it is threaded all over my home in things lent and learned and looked at every day. A photograph on my desk: Mum is gazing straight into the lens. Her eyes are lit with laughter, her expression warm, engaged. And I think: 'There she is! That's Mum.' It's like reaching for a lifebelt.

And I am afloat: I remember.

Epilogue

In those last days of her life, as she lay quiet and still in her bed facing the window, my mother said to me, 'I love you.'

'I love you too, Mum,' I said.

She took my hand in hers and she kissed my fingers.

'I love you so much,' she said again, before dozing off.

It was only in the days after she'd gone that it occurred to me: I never asked her who she thought I was then.

It didn't matter.

Acknowledgements

Books don't get onto anybody's shelves without a great agent, to read an early - and often clumsy - draft, to believe in what a writer is trying to say. Dotti Irving, of Greyhound Literary, read and re-read my words. She tempered my passion where it needed tempering. She helped me polish the manuscript where it needed polishing. And she was wonderful company in the process. Thank you, Dotti; this would not have seen the light of day without you. A big thank-you to everybody at Bedford Square Publishers - to Jamie Hodder-Williams for seeing timely merit in this, and to all the team; Polly Halsey, you were endlessly patient as I proofread again and again. Also, to my editor Sophie Lazur who helped me make my story watertight. Thank you to Emma Dowson at Emma Draude PR for encouragement and for helping to launch this.

Thank you to the newspaper editors over the years who helped me get my words out and especially those who encouraged my writing on dementia - Cathy Hilborn Feng at the *South China Morning Post* who commissioned my series, *Decoding Dementia*, and Damian Cullen at *The Irish Times* who commissioned a column. Readers' responses to those made me feel less alone on this journey and encouraged me to keep looking to the science.

Thanks to all the experts I have approached over the years in an effort to understand the brain, whether in mental illness, post stroke or, especially, Dementia. You were tolerant of my questions and patiently helped me understand the science as lay-language. Special thanks to Professor Craig Ritchie - Founder and CEO of Scottish Brain Sciences and Professor of Brain Health and Neurodegenerative Medicine at St Andrews University - who unwittingly gave me the title and read pages of extracts to make sure I'd translated the research accurately.

Thanks to Dr David Merrill at the Pacific Neuroscience Institute, whom I had several cross-continental zoom calls with at the wrong end of the day for him, and who also read pages of the manuscript. Thanks to Dr Dorina Cadar, Senior Lecturer in Cognitive Epidemiology and Dementia at Brighton and Sussex Medical School, whose expertise is sharpened by empathy; her father suffered too. Thanks also to Dr Malaz Boustani, geriatrician and neuroscientist at the Indiana University School of Medicine, Dr Albert Hofman Chair of the Department of Epidemiology at Harvard T H Chan School of Public Medicine, Andrew Sommerlad at University College London and Professor Yaakov Stern, Professor of Neuropsychology at Columbia University and to Andrew Lees, Professor of Neurology at the National Hospital for Neurology and Neurosurgery in London, for his encouragment as I began to write my own story about these Sepia Galactic Storms. All were generous with their time, again and again.

Heartfelt thanks to palliative care doctor, Kathryn Mannix, who responded to my desperate small-hours Instagram message in the middle of the night one night. She guided me through some of the most difficult hours of my life.

Thanks to seasoned writer, Sophy Roberts, who championed a newbie and pointed me in the right direction when I was floundering. Thank you to all the authors who have described Dementia accurately, powerfully, differently, for no two cases of this hideous illness present the same: Nicci Gerrard, Andrea Gillies, Sandeep Jauhar, Suzanne Finnamore and Octavia Bright; you learn a little from everybody's story. I read many.

Thanks to the wonderful Asina who calmly helped me carry Mum through her illness, metaphorically, with kindness, humour and wisdom, and literally when Mum became so disabled it took two of us to lift her.

Thanks to dear friends who made it easier to talk about a hard illness: to Eliza whom I leant on often, and who introduced herself to Mum again and again, and always with the grace of a first time; to my darling Caroline whom my mother loved until she forgot who she was and whom we lost to another brain illness - her regular and outrageous text messages made me laugh on the bleakest days. To Cathy whose medical background I relied on often, to Lesley whose rage when her own mother developed this disease matched my own, and to young Frieke, who was never afraid to help with Mum and never scared to ask questions. To be able to speak openly about this disease of the very old with the very young seemed hopeful.

Thank you to Marieke whose friendly and professional counsel was not just appreciated anyway but especially appreciated given my dislocated geography.

Thanks to my aunts and uncles on Mum's side: they often, after dad died, lent safe harbour. Mum's dear sister, Nora, and her husband David; Mum's brother, Pierce, with his wonderful Annie, helped us pick our way through the confusing fallout of her stroke; Mum's surviving sister, Trishi, whom she never forgot and who kept Mum's oldest memories safe, was ballast near the end in her wise counsel.

Thanks especially to my own siblings. My brother, Rob, for his always unruffled demeanour and excellent administration of our mother's affairs so that when I promised Mum her money was safe when she began to fret about it, I could confidently mean it. To my little sister, Carol, who put up with my tears, then made me laugh until I cried. We three have linked arms often in life as a united front - we did it again with Dementia. You need tight allies to face this disease; Rob and Carol were mine.

To my husband, Ant, whose practical good sense meant I made better plans and who surprised me with his intuition that to buy into the fiction conjured by Dementia was the right thing to do. To my precious, precious children, Ben, Amelia, Hattie, who remained stoic for me in the face of all this, despite watching a beloved last grandparent change beyond recognition to somebody who no longer recognised them. This was their loss too.

Thanks to Dad, who taught me that to know an illness, you must call it by its name, and that to understand it, you need to learn the language that describes it.

And finally, thanks to Mum. For gifting me words, for giving me courage. If only you could have read this, so that you knew. Perhaps you did anyway.

You all helped me to swim against the tide.

ABOUT THE AUTHOR

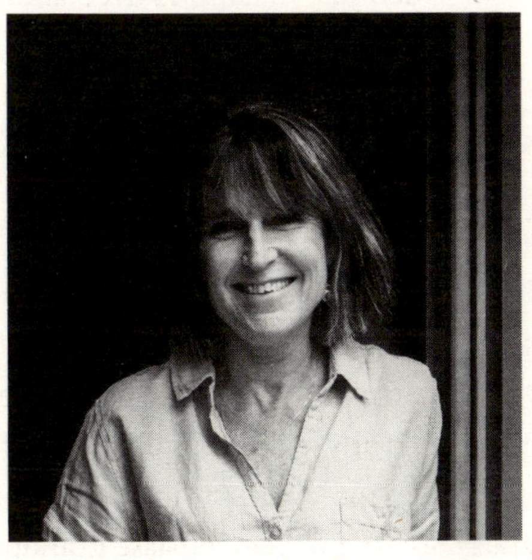

Anthea Rowan is a writer, journalist and blogger. She writes for newspapers and magazines across the world. She contributes to *Vogue*, the *Washington Post*, *The Irish Times* and the *South China Morning Post*. She lives in Africa. Mostly.

anthearowan.com

@Anthea_Rowan

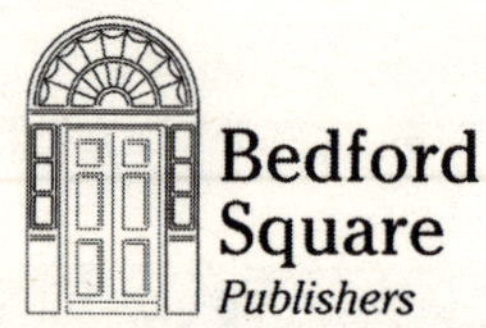

Bedford Square Publishers is an independent publisher of fiction and non-fiction, founded in 2022 in the historic streets of Bedford Square London and the sea mist shrouded green of Bedford Square Brighton.

Our goal is to discover irresistible stories and voices that illuminate our world.

We are passionate about connecting our authors to readers across the globe and our independence allows us to do this in original and nimble ways.

The team at Bedford Square Publishers has years of experience and we aim to use that knowledge and creative insight, alongside evolving technology, to reach the right readers for our books. From the ones who read a lot, to the ones who don't consider themselves readers, we aim to find those who will love our books and talk about them as much as we do.

We are hunting for vital new voices from all backgrounds – with books that take the reader to new places and transform perceptions of the world we live in.

Follow us on social media for the latest Bedford Square Publishers news.

@bedsqpublishers

facebook.com/bedfordsq.publishers

@bedfordsq.publishers

bedfordsquarepublishers.co.uk